OBSTETRICS AND GYNECOLOGY ADVANCES

OBSTETRIC AND GYNECOLOGY CASE REPORT

Obstetrics and Gynecology Advances

Additional books and e-books in this series can be found on Nova's website under the Series tab.

OBSTETRICS AND GYNECOLOGY ADVANCES

OBSTETRIC AND GYNECOLOGY CASE REPORT

DWIANA OCVIYANTI
EDITOR

nova
Medicine & Health
New York

Library of Congress Cataloging-in-Publication Data

Names: Ocviyanti, Dwiana, Faculty of Medicine Universitas Indonesia, Jakarta, Indonesia, editor. |
Title: Obstetric and Gynecology Case Report
Description: New York: Nova Science Publishers, [2019] | Series: Obstetrics and Gynecology Advances | Includes bibliographical references and index.
Identifiers: LCCN 2019954097 (print) | ISBN 9781536167115 (hardcover) |
ISBN 9781536167122 (adobe pdf)

Published by Nova Science Publishers, Inc. † New York

CONTENTS

PREFACE

This book entitled *Obstetrics and Gynecology Case Report* contains various cases in Obstetrics and Gynecology field. Twenty-six cases are included in this book chapter starting from rare cases to challenging cases.

The description and management of these cases are expected to be able to help specialists, general practitioners, and midwifes in dealing with similar cases. In addition there are also explanation about holistic management in several cases which are often found in daily practice.

We hope that this book can be useful in increasing knowledge and skill in obstetric and gynecology field. So that maternal and neonatal mortality can be reduce. In addition quality of life among women can be increased and improved.

Chapter 1 - The aim of this study was to assess the biological, psychological, and social aspects of *abortus provocatus*. A 17-year-old adolescent from Makassar, Indonesia, presented to Dr. Cipto Mangunkusumo Hospital with a chief complaint of a 4-month history of late menstruation. Although the patient was unaware that she was pregnant, the result of a pregnancy test was positive. The patient visited Dr. Cipto Mangunkusumo Hospital to avoid family and neighbors in Makassar. She was then diagnosed with late intrauterine fetal death of a singleton pregnancy at gestational week 18. From information obtained from her family, the patient's mother was angry and disappointed about the unplanned pregnancy. The patient denied having an abortion. Pregnancy is complicated by biopsychological and social factors, especially among adolescents. Termination of an unknown or unplanned pregnancy is considered a criminal act.

Chapter 2 - *Background*: Each year there are 15 million preterm babies born with a variety of survival chances. Preterm premature rupture of membranes (PPROM) represents one-third of preterm deliveries. Ruptured membranes before 24 weeks affect 0.4% of pregnancies, with mortality up to 70% reported in 2000. Preterm birth may cause high-risk impairments and places a heavy burden on families and the health system. Therefore, the termination of pregnancy has become an immediate proposal in cases of PPROM before 24 weeks.

Case Illustration: A women aged 25 years old was diagnosed as PPROM 14 days on primigravida at 19 weeks of gestation, singleton live fetus, with small amount of amniotic fluid. The patient was first treated conservatively with multivitamins and hydration for two weeks before they came to the Cipto Mangunkusumo Hospital. In our hospital, the patient and husband were educated regarding the poor prognosis associated with PPROM below 20 weeks and were advised to terminate the pregnancy. It was then decided to terminate the pregnancy. It was the first pregnancy for the patient, and it was expected to be the first grandchild for both parents of the patient. After delivery, both the patient and husband had a difficult time coping. PPROM impacts the biopsychosocial aspects of both maternal and neonates. Mothers might be at risk for systemic infection even after delivery, while newborn babies might be at high risk of respiratory distress syndrome, NEC, or prolonged intubation, which leads to stress and financial burden on the parents. The feelings of separation and exclusion with their baby could be related to the lack of physical and emotional closeness, which are essential factors in the early relationship between parents and their newborn infant. Mothers may also experience several and often conflicting emotional reactions, such as grief, sadness, guilt, fear, anger, loss of self-esteem, and sense of failure. Comprehensive education using a multidisciplinary approach is critical to have the best decisions from parents regarding pregnancy condition.

Conclusion: PPROM below 20 weeks likely negatively impacts the parent's physical, emotional, and socio-cultural aspects. Therefore, proper comprehensive education using a holistic approach must be given to reduce the negative impacts.

Chapter 3 - *Background*: Pregnancy among unmarried women is far more likely to be unintended and have negative effects. Women who carry unintended pregnancies are more likely to experience pregnancy-related problems, delayed antenatal care, adverse birth outcomes such as preterm birth and low birth weight, and adverse socioeconomic consequences, such as psychosocial stress and poor mental health.

Case Study: A 30-year-old woman presented at Dr. Cipto Mangunkusumo Hospital with premature rupture of amniotic membranes at 39 weeks of gestation. She had undergone a caesarian section. Both this pregnancy and her previous one were unintended, and she was unmarried during both.She had not received ANC at any public or private health services. The patient was afreelance worker and resided with her first child.

Discussion: Compared with pregnancies in married women, those among unmarried women tend to occur at a younger age among those with a lower educational level and among those who are unemployed or living in poverty. Women who experience unwanted pregnancies are 2.1 times more likely not to make maximum use of ANC care. Additionally, they are less motivated to seek information regarding the health of their pregnancies. The importance of preventing unintended pregnancies, especially in low economic status communities, can be achieved by health promotion and government prioritization of the screening of women with unintended pregnancies and implementation of the first thousand days of life program from Indonesia Minsitry of Health.

Conclusion: Unwanted pregnancies affect ANC behavior. The effect of unwanted pregnancy status varies according to the mother's economic status.

Chapter 4 - Reproductive health has attracted special attention since the topic was first raised at the International Conference on Population and Development in Cairo, Egypt, in 1994. At the conference, it was agreed to change the paradigm of managing population problems and development via control of population and fertility to focus on reproductive health and fulfillment of reproductive rights. Article 71 of Law Number 36 of 2009 concerning health states that reproductive health must consider biophysical, mental, and social aspects together and not merely as the condition of being free from disease or disability related to the system, functions, and reproductive process in males and females. We have reported Indonesian demographics regarding pregnant women, labor, and family planning until 2018.

Chapter 5 - Incest, a form of child sexual abuse, is a public health concern that has been commonly neglected and concealed. Factors such as inadequate communication skills to recognize the victim and the social inability to manage reports of suspected child sexual abuse may be responsible for this neglect. Global information may play a primary role in influencing sexual content. Victims' silence, and cultural and societal stigma exacerbate the problem. Pregnancy due to incest results in biopsychosocial impacts, thus creating a burden some global health problem. This paper explores a holistic approach from the biological, psychological, and social aspects of a *34*-week teenage pregnancy and intrauterine fetal death case.In the case illustrated in this paper, an 18-year-old pregnant woman was admitted to Cipto Mangunkusumo Hospital. She had suffered preterm labor when 34 weeks pregnant, which resulted in intrauterine fetal death. During the pregnancy, it was discovered that she had a history of forced sexual intercourse with her stepfather until she became pregnant. Her mother was too afraid to report it at first, but as her daughter's pregnancy progressed, the mother reported the matter and the father was eventually arrested. According to previous literature, family incest is rarely reported. Generally, children are the victims of rape; in particular, the perpetrators of this sexual violence are fathers and the victims, their daughters. Psychologically, sexual violence or rape destroys the mentality of the victim. Incest is rarely reported to the authorities because of the fear of tarnishing the family name and having a criminal record.

Chapter 6 - Incidence of tuberculosis in pregnancy is high worldwide with more than 200.000 active tuberculosis in pregnant woman at 2011, especially in Africa and South East Asia. Tuberculosis infection is caused by inhaled *M. tuberculosis* turn to be active or dormant state. Adequate antenatal care is very important. Newborn who has mother with active tuberculosis, both of them are treated. Mrs A, a 37 year old grandemultiparous woman presented at 34 weeks gestation with signs of premature labor. Upon presentation, she also developed cough, weight loss, night sweats. Chest X-ray showed bilateral infiltrate pattern, suggestive of tuberculosis. She had normal delivery at term pregnancy, delivering a small baby and rooming in with the mother. After finding and diagnosis tuberculosis this patient from clinical and chest X-ray examination, she received one month treatment for tuberculosis and plan to receive a total six months treatment. The baby also got prophylaxis Izoniazide (INH) for 6 months. Tuberculosis infection in baby must be ruled out, and baby should be given isoniazid preventive therapy, followed by BCG vaccination after 2 weeks of treatment and negative skin test. Management of tuberculosis during pregnancy not only from biological approach but also include psychosocial approach. The management should be integrated among medical specialty, public health care, government, and patient itself.

Chapter 7 - Cesarean scar pregnancy (CSP) is a rare case that occurred when the embryo implants to the wall of myometrium in previous caesarean scar. The condition is a serious condition due to the several consequences. A standard treatment protocol for this condition has not yet been established due to the limitation of data. This case report describes a patient who was diagnosed with a CSP at 12 weeks of gestation with beta-human chorionic gonadotropin (β-hcG) levels of 34,968.12 mIU/mL. She was successfully treated with systemic methotrexate followed by evacuation through a hysteroscopic procedure using an Integrated Bigatti Shaver. This report adds to the literature on safe and effective treatments for CSP. A 35-year-old, gravida 4, para 3, woman with a history of two prior term cesarean sections was diagnosed with a CSP during a routine first-trimester ultrasound at 12 weeks of gestation. She had reported spotting in the previous 2 weeks. Ultrasound revealed a gestational sac with a diameter of 2.62 cm. Methotrexate 50 mg/m^2 was administered as a single dose via intravenous infusion according to the "two-dose regimen," following which β-hcG levels decreased. The present case is an important contribution to the research on

CSP treatment. Systemic methotrexate followed by a hysteroscopic procedure is a safe and effective approach for conservative treatment of a first-trimester CSP while preserving fertility.

Chapter 8 – *Background*: Based on a population survey conducted in 2015, the maternal mortality rate in Indonesia was 305 per 100,000 live births. Hence, holistic management is needed to reduce maternal and infant mortality to achieve the target set as part of Sustainable Development Goals. Aside from comprehensive and accurate management, clinicians should propose a management strategy that involves an interprofessional approach to manage the patients optimally.

Aim: This study aims to discuss holistic management in obstetric patients who require interprofessional management based on their biopsychosocial aspects.

Method: This case series reported 19 patients with an obstetric issue who were admitted to Dr. Cipto Mangunkusumo General Hospital in 2018-2019. The inclusion criterion is obstetric cases that emphasize biopsychosocial management.

Result: In 2018-2019, we encountered 7 cases of adolescent pregnancy, 2 cases of preeclampsia, 3 cases of preterm labor, 2 cases of abortion on unwanted pregnancy, 1 case of unwanted pregnancy with carcinoma on chemoradiation, 1 case of wanting pregnancy during an end-stage disease, 1 case of pregnancy on neglected people, and 1 case of unwanted pregnancy because of economic problem.

Conclusion: Holistic and comprehensive management are needed for obstetric patients to reduce maternal and infant mortality. Holistic management included biopsychosocial aspect.

Chapter 9 - *Introduction*: Autoimmune hepatitis (AIH) is a chronic inflammatory disease characterized by progressive hepatocellular inflammation not related to alcohol consumption, viral infection, exposure to hepatotoxic drugs, or genetic liver disorders. AIH is associated with a high rate of miscarriage, stillbirth, and premature delivery. This study aimed to discuss the optimal management of AIH during pregnancy in order to maintain the pregnancy up to term. We also determined whether pregnancy influences the flare-up of AIH or vice versa and what the best treatment for AIH during pregnancy is.

Case Illustration: A 32-year-old pregnant woman diagnosed with AIH delivered a healthy baby vaginally at 38 weeks of gestational age.

Discussion: The treatment strategy for AIH is to obtain complete remission and avoid further progression of the disease. The European Association for the Study of the Liver (EASL) states that the first-line therapy for AIH is prednisone/prednisolone, followed by the addition of azathioprine after 2 weeks.

Conclusion: Optimal management of AIH during pregnancy is required in order to maintain the pregnancy up to term.

Chapter 10 - The progestin-only subdermal implant levonorgestrel is a very effective contraceptive with a failure rate of only 0.05% within the first year of typical use. We herein present the case of a patients with two-rod levonorgestrel failure after discontinuing anti-tuberculosis medication at a district hospital. A 24-year-old female, para 1, was referred to the obstetrics polyclinic due to a positive pregnancy test. She had a two-rod levonorgestrel implant (Indoplant©) for the last two years. Seven months before referral, she was treated with rifampicinfor 5 months due to suspicious tuberculous lymphadenitis. An intrauterine pregnancy of 8^{+1} weeks with a crown-rump length of 1.72 mm was identified, and the implant was removed. Discussion: Rifampicin is known to induce liver CYP3A4 and decrease the area under the concentration-time curve by 55% for the mechanism of action from levonogestrel. Concomitant use of rifampicin can reduce contraceptive agent concentrations, increasing pregnancy risk. The recommendation in these patients is pregnancy continuation because the implant does not affect the progression of pregnancy.

Chapter 11 - Embryo Quality after Intra-cytoplasmic Sperm Injection Involving Sperm Associated with Azoospermia and Aged Oocytes: A Case Report Embryo quality determines the pregnancy rate and development of healthy offspring. Embryo profiling can help determine embryo quality through qualification and quantification of various parameters. Here we report a case of successful fertilization with intra-cytoplasmic sperm injection (ICSI) involving sperm associated with azoospermia and aged oocytes. Studies have reported success of ICSI involving sperm associated with azoospermia and aged oocytes, and the findings of the present report will fill the literature gap by providing evidence on the fertilization success rate with ICSI involving sperm associated with azoospermia. A 39-year-old man and 35-year-old woman visited our infertility center. ICSI was performed, and embryos were obtained. Two embryos were freshly transferred on day 3, and two embryos were frozen. As the fresh embryo transfer failed, the frozen embryos were used for frozen embryo transfer, and pregnancy was successfully achieved. We believe that the DNA quality of the testicular sperm determines the pregnancy success rate. Although moderate-quality embryos in frozen embryo transfer were exposed to freezing effects, pregnancy was successfully achieved, possibly because of better receptivity of the endometrium.

Chapter 12 - During *in vitro* fertilization (IVF), an egg is fertilized by sperm outside the body (coined as *in vitro*). It is most indicated when infertility results from one or more causes having no other effective treatments, and it is often the best treatment for couples with multifactor infertility because it can address or overcome all contributing causes at the same time. Concurrent with an IVF cycle, cellular biopsies can be obtained from a developing embryo for genetic evaluation. A screening approach is preimplantation genetic screening (PGS), which is used to evaluate embryos for chromosomal abnormalities. We present the case of a 38-year-old woman who had undergone two intrauterine insemination procedures and three IVF procedures previously but did not become pregnant. Her body mass index was 20.4 kg/m^2, and gynecological findings were normal. Transvaginal ultrasound examination revealed that the uterus was in anteflexion, with a normal size and shape, the endometrium was regular at 9 mm; moreover, both ovaries showed a normal size. She received ovarian stimulation with a total recombinant follicle-stimulating hormone at a dose of 3300 IU. Oocyte retrieval was performed, and seven oocytes were obtained. Eventually, three were fertilized and two embryos were frozen. PGS was performed, which revealed that one embryo was normal and one had aneuploidy. Single embryo transfer was performed, and she successfully became pregnant. Morphologically normal-looking embryos can harbor genetic or epigenetic defects. PGS appears to play an important role in the identification of the best embryo for transfer.

Chapter 13 - *Background*: Infertility is associated with psychological problems being experienced by both partners, and in vitro fertilization (IVF) is one of many infertility treatment procedures. IVF significantly influences patients and their family's psychology. This report reviews the biopsychosocial aspects of infertility in relation to recurrent IVF failure.

Case Illustration: A 42-year-old female patient with primary infertility for the past 16 years requested consultation on pregnancy programs. She had a history of cystectomy surgery for endometriotic cysts. At presentation, there were no problems with the husband's sperm quality, the patient had undergone three failed insemination attempts, followed by three failed IVF attempts. Ultrasound examination found left tubal enlargement size $25 \times 13 \times 16$ mm^3, correspond to hydrosalpinx. The patient was also diagnosed as having diminished ovarian reserves. She underwent a hysteroscopy with subsequent laparoscopy for endometriosis in the left fallopian tube, which resulted in a left-sided salpingectomy. After laparoscopic surgery, the patient plans to undergo one final IVF procedure.

Discussion: After failed IVF cycles, women experience an increase in depressive symptoms with lower levels of self-esteem, compared to those before the treatment cycle. A problem-solving coping strategy is associated with better psychological adjustment, whereas the use of avoidance coping and social isolation has the opposite effect; hence, behavioral strategies may help these patients deal with their loss of control.

Conclusion: This case illustrates the association between infertility and ART failure and its biopsychosocial implications that require appropriate support to reduce patient distress, help patients come to terms with their situation, and facilitate decision making.

Chapter 14 - Polycystic ovary syndrome (PCOS) is commonly observed in women of reproductive age. This syndrome presents with symptoms such as amenorrhea, hirsutism, and obesity. Impairment of feedback between the hypothalamus–pituitary axis and ovary increases the secretion of estrogen, decreasing the secretion of follicle-stimulating hormone (FSH). Herein, we report the case of a 29-year-old married women who sought fertility consultation at our intuition. The following laboratory results were obtained: an elevated luteinizing hormone (LH) level during the follicular stage (22.390 mIU/mL) and an FSH/LH ratio of 4.6 (elevated >2.5). Such findings are indicative of PCOS. Moreover, the patient presented with amenorrhea and irregular menstruation. Her last menstrual period was 1.5 years back. The patient has been experiencing primary infertility for 3 years. Ultrasonography revealed the following results: retroflexion on the cavum uteri, uterus of normal size, endometrial thickness of 11 mm, and polycystic ovaries.

Chapter 15 - Aggressive management of endometrial cancer often involves hysterectomy, a procedure where a part of the uterus is taken out to eliminate the cancer. This procedure results in secondary infertility and this may cause significant morbidity, especially in patients who wishes to have children. A 29-year-old woman presented with a chief complaint of vaginal bleeding. Curettage and hysteroscopy revealed a low-risk endometrial cancer. The patient was first given conservative therapy to preserve the uterus. After 1 year of treatment, her condition did not improve. The patient was of low socioeconomic status and was unable to afford *in vitro* fertilization. She decided to undergo hysterectomy, even though she was of childbearing age. Secondary infertility due to medical procedures significantly impacts the patient's biology, psychology, and social factors. This patient's decision to undergo aggressive treatment for endometrial cancer is influenced by her disadvantaged background. A patient's socioeconomic status influences her decision making and affects her quality of life. This case illustrates how a patient's socioeconomic status influences clinical decision making and progression of the disease. The clinician must appreciate socioeconomic factors that may influence a patient's preference in managing endometrial cancer.

Chapter 16 - The presence of normal endometrial mucosa outside of the uterine cavity known as endometriosis. Endometriosis patients complain of several symptoms, including chronic pelvic pain in 50% of patients, subfertility in 30–50%, and dysmenorrhea in 12–32%. Chronic pain and subfertility can affect the psychological status of endometriosis patients. Adequate counseling can improve the patients' and their spouses' acceptance of the condition and improve treatment compliance.A 31-year-old woman presented withchief complaints of dysmenorrhea with a VAS score of 6, anemia due to abnormal uterine bleeding, and primary infertility for six years. The patient had suffered from pelvic pain for 10 years. She used to work but resigned because of her condition. She also admitted that the symptoms affect her daily activity and social life. The subfertility causes her to avoid meeting friends and family.The physical examination and ultrasound identified adenomyosis and a right endometriosis cyst. The patient was hospitalized for transfusion and given an analgetic and dienogest. Dysmenorrhea had affected the patient's daily activities for approximately 10 years and had worsened in the past two years. She received medical treatment, and the pain decreased. However, she had not been regularly taking her medication recently, and she returned to the hospital because of abnormal uterine bleeding and pain. The management for endometriosis is to relief the symptom and increase the chance for fertility. Psychologically, the pain and the frequent admissions to the hospital affected her life, causing depression and eliminating her social life. Adequate counseling provided to the patient and her husband regarding her condition and understanding the possibility of treatment for pain and infertility may decrease the psychological problem.

Chapter 17 - The disorder of sex development (DSD) is defined as the congenital conditions in which the development of the chromosomal, gonadal, or anatomical sex is atypical. Congenital adrenal hyperplasia (CAH) consists of a family of disorders caused by reduced activity of enzymes required for the biosynthesis of cortisol in the adrenal cortex, resulting in increased levels of dehydroepiandrosterone sulfate and testosterone. The masculinization of a DSD 46XX patient with CAH is caused by excessive levels of male hormones. During adolescence, the diagnosis of DSD is often an alarming and traumatic event for both the adolescent and the family, considering that this a rare disorder and absolutely foreign to the majority of non-medical individuals. The management of DSD is extraordinarily heterogeneous across centers, and pre- and post-treatment evaluations are mostly subjective, examiner-dependent, and influenced by cultural norms. In this article, we report a rare case of delayed diagnosis of DSD 46XX in a 23-year-old patient with CAH. The patient exhibiting genital ambiguity and primary amenorrhea, desired to be a male person. The levels of hormones were as follows: high dehydroepiandrosterone sulfate, 937.8 μg/dL); high testosterone, 27.3 nmL/L; and low estradiol, 45 pg/mL, corresponding to the normal levels of a male. A multidisciplinary team, consisting of a reproductive endocrinologist, plastic surgeon, metabolic endocrinologist, psychiatrist, and the hospital ethics committee, collaborated to address the patient's desire regarding her gender condition. Prolonged exposure to androgens results in masculinization of the brain. Therefore, she preferred to become a male instead of a female. She underwent total laparoscopy hysterectomy and masculinizing reconstructive surgery on her external genitalia. In addition, prior to and following surgery, the patient received psycho-adaptive therapy.

Chapter 18 - Fallopian tube cancer (FTC) is one of the most rare malignancies of the female reproductive system, accounting for only 0.14%–1.8% of all gynecologic cancers. Its rarity contributes to the difficulty in making a definite diagnosis and determining its prognosis, and its diagnosis is rarely done preoperatively. The presence of a hydrosalpinx is a hallmark of FTC. Here, we report three cases of FTC to explore an approach for its diagnosis and management. Because FTC shares similar clinical findings with ovarian carcinoma, it is often diagnosed intraoperatively. The elevation of serum CA125 levels contributes to the diagnosis of FTC. Surgical cytoreduction followed by chemotherapy is the best therapeutic option for FTC.

Chapter 19 - Fallopian tube carcinoma (FTC) is one of the rarest malignancies of female reproductive system, accounting for only 0.14%–1.8% of all gynecological cancers. Establishing a clear diagnosis and prognosis of FTC are generally considered difficult. In this study, we aimed to determine the histopathology of FTC and to determine the correlation between its histopathological and clinical findings. A 54-year-old unmarried woman presented with nausea, vomiting, and abdominal pain since 1 month prior to admission. She was diagnosed with suspected ovarian carcinoma with pleural effusions based on clinical and tumor marker tests and imaging. Accordingly, exploratory laparotomy was performed, and ascites and enlarged fallopian tubes that adhered to the rectosigmoid were noted. Subsequently, she underwent total hysterectomy, bilateral salpingo-oophorectomy, omentectomy, peritoneal biopsy, and loop sigmoid colostomy because of the adhesion. Pathological analysis revealed high-grade serous carcinoma in both fallopian tubes and ovaries. Furthermore, pleural fluid cytology showed positive results for a metastatic tumor. Thus, six cycles of docetaxel–carboplatin chemotherapy were administered. Primary FTC is a rare gynecological malignancy. Serous FTC resembles the tumors of its ovarian counterparts with papillae, cellular buds, slit-like glandular spaces, solid sheets, and occasionally tumor giant cells and psammoma bodies.

Chapter 20 - Cervical fibroids are one of the most interesting findings in fibroid cases owing to their location relative to other important structures. In cases involving a large cervical fibroid, the symptoms are mostly related to anterior and posterior mechanical pressures from the fibroid. Thus, the management should be aimed at releasing these pressures by removing the mass through myomectomy or hysterectomy. Considering the high risk of bladder and bowel injury, these procedures should be precisely performed with advanced understanding of anatomical alterations related to the fibroid. We report a case of a large cervical fibroid in a patient with a history of laparotomy exploration. In this case, we were unable to perform hysterectomy due to severe adhesion. The patient was a 40-year-old female with concomitant endometriosis. Subsequently, a gonadotropin-releasing hormone agonist was administered and the patient was referred to our hospital. We performed relaparotomy hysterectomy, and the cervical fibroid was completely removed. Notably, the bladder and bowel remained intact without other complications.

Chapter 21 - Cervical cancer most commonly recurs in the parametrium, pelvic lymph nodes, and vagina. The incidence of incisional skin metastasis from cervical cancer is extremely rare and usually results in a poor prognosis. A 54-year-old female patient was referred with an abdominal mass after definitive treatment for cervical cancer. Fourteen months before admission, she underwent radical hysterectomy with bilateral salpingo-oophorectomy and pelvic lymphadenectomy. Her abdominal examination at presentation revealed a 2 cm diameter mobile mass with solid consistency. Her fine needle aspiration biopsy results were positive for metastatic carcinoma. The patient was then given chemotherapy, at the end of which the mass still existed. We then performed wide excision of the mass followed by re-radiation therapy. Metastasis of the incisional site after definitive therapy for cervical cancer is an extremely rare occurrence in the follow-up of tumor patients and represents a challenge for the interdisciplinary team. Factors that affect the recurrence time, optimal management, and prognosis in these cases must be further studied.

Chapter 22 - *Objective*: To determine the diagnostic modality and therapeutic management of malignant vaginal melanomas.

Method: Evidence-based case report and review, with literature from the PubMed and Cochrane databases.

Results: We identified 36 studies, of which seven could be evaluated. One serial case report concluded that melanoma should be diagnosed histopathologically and treated with local resection as the primary treatment, followed by chemotherapy as an adjuvant therapy; a median survival of 419 days post-therapy was reported. One systematic review did not identify significant differences in survival time after radical excision compared with wide local excision (WLE) (median 33 vs. 19 months, P = 0.065). Four studies concluded that wide excisions with thorough removal of the macroscopic tumor and negative-free margins have better survival rates thantreatment with primary radiotherapy, and inadvanced-stage melanoma cases, palliative chemotherapy is preferred.

Conclusion: In any patient with suspected vaginal melanoma, diagnosis should be established by histopathological examination, and staging should be determined based on pelvic examination and radiology work-up.All patients with vaginal cancer should be referred to and treated by a multidisciplinary gynecological oncology team, withWLE as the recommended treatment and chemotherapy and radiation for unresectable cases. Palliative chemoradiation should be considered for advanced-stage disease.

Chapter 23 - The diagnosis of labial fusion is sometimes difficult. Total closure of the vaginal opening because of dense adhesion can be misdiagnosed as congenital urogenital sinus or Mullerian anomaly. An incorrect diagnosis mayresult in the patient receiving wrong information and an inappropriate treatment. Here wereport a case of labial fusion in a 34-year-old woman. She was referred with an initial diagnosis of congenital urogenital sinus anomaly (low vaginal septum). On history taking, she mentioned frequent vulvar erosion during bicycle riding in her adolescence. On physical examination, total labial fusion was noted, with only a pinpoint hole. Additionally, on ultrasound, all structures at the vulvo-vaginal area could be distinguished. Thus, a final diagnosis of labial fusion was made. She underwent appropriate surgery without any complications. In such cases, careful history taking, physical examination, and transrectal ultrasound imaging can help make an accurate diagnosis of labial fusion and help patient achieve appropriate management to relieveall the symptoms.

Chapter 24 - Extramammary Paget's disease is rare malignant neoplasm occur in women. It arises from apocrine glan-bearing skin cells or manifestation of adjacent primary anal, rectal or bladder adenocarcinoma. A visible lesion is typically erythematous plaque occur in external genitalia, which mimicking dermatology lesions. However due to its slow growing, it may cause delayed diagnosis then consequently worsen prognosis. Here we present case of 46 yo woman with persistent reddish plaque in vulvar area for 1 year. The lesion was mimicking fungal infection that she received the treatment from dermatologist. Biopsy result was extramammary Paget's disease. Patient was received further biopsy lesion to determine malignant area then continue with wide local excision with keystone flap. Till this day, patient has routinely control to plastic surgeon clinic for further wound care.

Chapter 25 – *Background*: Several patients are referred to Dr.Cipto Mangunkusumo National General Hospital due to complicated gynecological problems, both biological and psychological, which affect their life. Therefore, a holistic biopsychosocial treatment should be implemented, which requires interprofessional cooperation.

Aim: To present gynecological cases requiring holistic treatment and interprofessional management

Method: Seven patients with gynecological problems were admitted to Ciptomangunkusumo General Hospital during 2018–2019. The inclusion criteria were gynecological conditions requiring holistic management.

Result: Of the seven patients, three had endometriosis, one had adenomyosis, one had Mayer–Rokitansky–Küster–Hauser syndrome, one had fistule vesicovaginal, and one had experienced sexual abuse. These patients were managed in collaboration with other professionals, including pediatricians, psychiatrists, and law experts. Moreover, the patient's family should also be involved in patient management.

Conclusion: In complicated gynecological cases with a high difficulty level, holistic management plays an important role in treatment. An interprofessional approach also plays an important role to increase patients' quality of life.

Chapter 26 - *Background*: Only a few cases of cervical tuberculosis were reported in the literature, making it a rare condition. Additionally, the history and cervical characteristics of cervical tuberculosis resemble those of invasive cervical cancer.

Case report: A 31-year-old nulliparous woman complained of having vaginal discharge and post-coital bleeding for 1 year prior to admission. The cervical examination revealed an irregular and fragile cervical mass that bled easily. The Pap smear test also suggests atypical squamous cell cannot exclude high-grade squamous intraepithelial lesion (ASCH). A suspected cervical cancer mass was visualized on our colposcopy view. A cervical mass biopsy revealed a chronic granulomatous cervicitis that is probably caused by tuberculous infection. Additionally, the serum interferon-gamma release assay (IGRA) test was positive. Therefore, the patient's clinical and histopathologic diagnosis was cervical tuberculosis. A 4-week administration of first-line antituberculosis treatment resulted in the improvement of the cervical lesion.

Conclusion: Based on the clinical and histopathological findings, our patient was diagnosed with cervical tuberculosis. First-line antituberculosis drugs are the treatment of choice for cervical tuberculosis.

SECTION 1: OBSTETRIC

In: Obstetric and Gynecology Case Report ISBN: 978-1-53616-711-5
Editor: Dwiana Ocviyanti

Chapter 1

A CASE OF ILLEGAL PREGNANCY TERMINATION BY AN ADOLESCENT GIRL

Ariel Timy** *and Dwiana Ocviyanti
Department of Obstetric and Gynecology, Faculty of Medicine, Universitas Indonesia, Dr. Cipto Mangunkusumo Hospital, Jakarta, Indonesia

ABSTRACT

The aim of this study was to assess the biological, psychological, and social aspects of *abortus provocatus*. A 17-year-old adolescent from Makassar, Indonesia, presented to Dr. Cipto Mangunkusumo Hospital with a chief complaint of a 4-month history of late menstruation. Although the patient was unaware that she was pregnant, the result of a pregnancy test was positive. The patient visited Dr. Cipto Mangunkusumo Hospital to avoid family and neighbors in Makassar. She was then diagnosed with late intrauterine fetal death of a singleton pregnancy at gestational week 18. From information obtained from her family, the patient's mother was angry and disappointed about the unplanned pregnancy. The patient denied having an abortion. Pregnancy is complicated by biopsychological and

* Corresponding Author's E-mail: arieltimy19@gmail.com.

social factors, especially among adolescents. Termination of an unknown or unplanned pregnancy is considered a criminal act.

Keywords: adolescent pregnancy, abortus provocatus

Introduction

Adolescent pregnancy is defined as the pregnancy of a female who is younger than 19 years. Various biopsychosocial aspects have significant effects on pregnancy. According to the United Nations Department of Economic and Social Affairs, 2010, Indonesia is one of 37 countries with a high percentage of young marriages and is the second highest in Southeast Asia after Cambodia [1]. Marriage at a young age is complicated by insufficient readiness in terms of mental and emotional health, education, and socio-economic status. Adolescent pregnancy, especially when unexpected, is associated with an increased incidence of abortion or *abortus provocatus*, even though abortion is considered illegal [2]. According to Indonesian law, abortion is defined as an evacuation of conception at any stage of development before 38–40 weeks of gestation [3]. In the United States, nearly half (49%) of the pregnancies were unintended in 2006. The rate of unintended pregnancy increased from 50 per 1000 women aged 15–44 years in 2001 to 52 in 2006 [4]. In England in 2010, there were 225,600 unintended pregnancies and 155,500 induced abortions [5]. The most common emotional reactions after pregnancy termination are relief, transient guilt, sadness, and a sense of loss [6].

Case Illustration

A 17-year-old unmarried Muslim female, who was a third-year high school student in the city of Makassar and living with her parents, presented to the maternity ward of Dr. Cipto Mangun Kusumo Hospital (Jakarta, Indonesia) with a chief complaint of a 4-month history of late menstruation

The patient was the youngest of three siblings born to a father who is an entrepreneur in the printing business and a mother who is a housewife. The patient reported that her last menstrual period ended on September 3, 2018. Although she denied being pregnant, the result of a pregnancy test was positive. The patient claimed to have had unprotected sex with her partner on two occasions and admitted to consuming medication for menstrual pain 1 month prior and an unknown herbal medicine 1 week prior to admission based on advice from her friends. She reported the loss of amniotic fluid, bleeding, and nausea over the last week. Due to the death of the fetus, the patient was referred to Dr. Cipto Mangunkusumo Hospital.

Upon admission, the patient's blood pressure was 110/70 mmHg with a pulse rate of 84 beats per minute, and respiration rate of 20 breaths per minute. On physical examination, no abnormalities were found. On an obstetric examination, the vulva and urethra were smooth with no active bleeding. Speculum examination revealed slippery portio, cervical ostium opening of 2 cm, visible tissue in portio, fluor negative, and fluxus positive. On vaginal toucher examination: soft portio, axial, 2 cm thick, 2 cm opening, and palpable tissue in portio.

Ultrasound examination revealed the presence of an intrauterine single fetus with no fetal heart rate, undetermined crown-rump length, negative Spalding sign, and no amniotic fluid. The patient was diagnosed with incipient abortion in G1, gestational week 18, late intrauterine fetal death, adolescent pregnancy, and unwanted pregnancy. Management of this patient included induction of 200 μg of vaginal misoprostol every 6 h, intravenous injection of 5 g of ampicillin/sulbactam, once per day for 4 days, and psychiatric and medico-legal forensics consultation. According to the medico-legal forensic consultation, the patient was suspected of inducing an abortion. Based on the results of the psychiatry consultation, the patient consumed an herbal medicine 1 week prior to admission with the intention of inducing an abortion. The patient admitted to unprotected sexual contact with her partner on two occasions around September of October of 2018. There was no history of threats, physical violence, or providing food/drink. According to the forensics examination, an incipient abortion in G1, gestational week 18, was suspected to be an *abortus provocatus*. Medical management recommendations were made by the Midwifery Department and the incidence was reported to the police. From the results of the psychiatric consultation, the patient was relieved that she was no longer pregnant. The patient claimed that she did not know that she was pregnant and only found out after being told by her mother 4 days prior to presentation. The patient admitted to having sex with her partner, who was 2 years older on two occasions. The patient commented that she felt sad and disappointed with her partner, but had intended to forgive him. The patient said that she was scared about possibly being pregnant. The patient and her parents wished to immediately terminate the pregnancy. The patient's parents expressed sadness and disappointment about their only daughter's experience because they wanted her to finish high school, as both had only completed junior high school. The mental status of the patient was consistent with that of an adolescent female, but she was less cooperative and resistant, while her psychomotor behavior was calm, but seemed to be guarded. Her speech was less than spontaneous, with sufficient volume and clear articulation. Her mood was dysphoric, limited, and harmonious with a coherent thought process and good perception. Supportive psychotherapy (empathy validation, reassurance) was recommended.

DISCUSSION

Adolescent pregnancy is often an undesirable situation for obvious reasons. However, the termination of a pregnancy or *abortus provocatus* is technically illegal under the Criminal Code of Indonesia [2, 7]. Pregnancy in adolescence is influenced by several factors, such as poor parental supervision, familial disappointment, environmental factors, and advances in communication technology with easy access pornography [2, 8]. The biopsychosocial concept is a medical approach from the perspectives of behavior, intellectual capacity, and psychological and social health.

Biological Aspects

Adolescent pregnancy is associated with a relatively greater prevalence of complications for both the mother and fetus. In this case, the complications were more toward the psychological and social aspects of the patient due to shame perceived by the patient, her family, and community. Psychologically, adolescents with premarital pregnancies will feel depressed, scared, confused, and embarrassed, which may increase the desire for an abortion. Moreover, women with an unwanted pregnancy may seek to have an abortion clandestinely, although such procedures can be unsafe when performed by an incompetent person, such as a "*dukun*." The complications of abortion include bleeding, infections, and even death [9].

Psychological Aspects

The psychological factors associated with adolescent pregnancy include: (i) a lack of parental guidance, as the roles of parents greatly influence the mental and psychological development of children, and those who are not content with familial relationships will tend to seek peace outside of the family; (ii) a lack of sex education, as about 65% of adolescents reported receiving information about sex from friends and 35% from pornographic films, while only 5% receive information from parents; and (iii) the development of communications technology, which can hinder mental development [8].

The advancement of science and technology had made it easier for teenagers to obtain information about sex. Adolescents who are pregnant outside of marriage face a variety of psychological problems, especially fear, disappointment, regret, and low self-esteem, which may result in efforts to eliminate the pregnancy by way of abortion. An abortion may be viewed as a smaller loss than continuing the pregnancy, as the situation becomes more complicated if the male partner does not acknowledge responsibility and leaves the female to fend for herself. In addition, the family may face difficulties in the community for the failure to provide moral education to their daughters. Under such circumstances, the woman may seek to have an abortion, which is considered a criminal act in Indonesia. Following abortion, the woman may have feelings of guilt and experience major depression, frustration, and emptiness. Post-abortion syndrome is characterized by the loss of self-esteem, nightmares, inability to enjoy sexual relations, hysterics, use of drugs, and suicide [10, 11].

Social Aspects

Adolescent pregnancy can also result in a number of social effects, such as criminal acts, as abortion is illegal in Indonesia, embarrassment to the woman and her family, negative impacts on education, economic hardship, and isolation from friends [3, 10, 12]. According to the Criminal Code of Indonesia, a woman who purposely performs an abortion or takes action to terminate the pregnancy in utero, or asks another to perform the procedure can be imprisoned for a period of up to 4 years [13, 14]. Strategies to address social problems associated with adolescent pregnancy need to involve joint interventions in education, skill development, and clinical and social support for adolescent mothers [3].

Conclusion

Adolescent pregnancy is associated with complex biopsychosocial problems, especially if the pregnancy is unwanted. We experienced a case of *abortus provocatus*, which is unsafe and can be fatal to the mother. Therefore, supervision in adolescent pregnancy is very important. In addition to health and medical aspects, supervision also includes social and psychological support to optimize conditions for pregnant adolescents.

REFERENCES

[1] Ministry of Health, Republic Indonesia. (2014). *Situasi Kesehatan Reproduksi Remaja.* [*Adolescent Reproductive Health Situation*]. Jakarta: Ministry of Health, Republic of Indonesia.

[2] Shaw, M., Lawlor, D.A., Najman, J.M., (2006). Teenage children of teenage mothers: Psychological, behavioural and health outcomes from an Australian prospective longitudinal study. *Soc. Sci. Med,* 62: 2526-2539.

[3] Ekotama S., Pudjiarto H., & Widiartana G. (2001). *Abortus provokatusbagi korban perkosaan: perspektif viktimologi kriminologi dan hukum pidana* [*Abortion provokatus for victims of rape: criminological perspective of criminology and criminical law*]. Yogyakarta: Universitas Atma Jaya Yogyakarta.

[4] Finer L.B., Zolna M.R., (2011). Unintended pregnancy in the United States: incidence and disparities 2006. *Contraception*, 84: 478-485.

[5] Montouchet, C., Trussell, J. (2013). Unintended pregnancies in England in 2010: costs to the National Health Service (NHS). *Contraception,* 87:149-153.

[6] Stotland. N. L. (1992). The myth of the abortion trauma syndrome. *JAMA,* 268:2078-2079.

[7] Azevedo, W.F., Diniz, M.B., Fonseca, E.S., Azevedo, L.M., Evangelista, C.B. 2015. Complications in adolescent pregnancy: Systematic review of the literature. *Einstein (Sao Paulo),* 13(4): 618-626.

[8] World Health Organization. (2018). *Adolescents: Health risks and solutions.*

[9] Cameron, S., Glasier, A., Lohr, P.A., Moreau, C., Munk-Olsen, T. (2017). Induced abortion, ESHRE Capri Workshop Group, *Human reproduction,* 32(6): 1160-1169.

[10] Hodgkinson, S., Beers, L., Southammakosane, C., Lewin, A. (2014). Addressing the mental health needs of pregnant and parenting adolescents. *Pediatrics,* 133(1):114-122.

[11] Patch, L.K., (1990). Adolescent pregnancy: Psychosocial issues. *Indiana Med,* 83(1), 30-33.

[12] Cook, S.M.C., Cameron, S.T. (2015). Social issues of teenage pregnancy. *Obstetr.Gynaecol.Rep.Med,* 25(9): 243-248.

[13] Hamzah, A. (1984). *Kitab undang-undang hukum pidana* [Book of criminal constitution law]. *Ghalia Indonesia*.

[14] Hanafiah, M.J. & Amir A. (1999). *Etika kedokteran & hukum kesehatan* [*Medical ethics and law*]. *EGC*.

In: Obstetric and Gynecology Case Report
Editor: Dwiana Ocviyanti
ISBN: 978-1-53616-711-5

Chapter 2

BIOPHYSICOSOCIAL IMPACTS ON PRETERM PREMATURE OF RUPTURED MEMBRANE (PPROM) BELOW 20 WEEKS

Bella Aprilia[1,*] and Dwiana Ocviyanti[2]
[1]Faculty of Medicine, Universitas Indonesia, Jakarta, Indonesia
[2]Department of Obstetric and Gynecology, Faculty of Medicine, Universitas Indonesia, Dr. Cipto Mangunkusumo Hospital, Jakarta, Indonesia

ABSTRACT

Each year there are 15 million preterm babies born with a variety of survival chances. Preterm premature rupture of membranes (PPROM) represents one-third of preterm deliveries. Ruptured membranes before 24 weeks affect 0.4% of pregnancies, with mortality up to 70% reported in 2000. Preterm birth may cause high-risk impairments and places a heavy burden on families and the health system. Therefore, the termination of pregnancy has become an immediate proposal in cases of PPROM before

* Corresponding Author's E-mail: bellaraphael.md@gmail.com.

24 weeks. A women aged 25 years old was diagnosed as PPROM 14 days on primigravida at 19 weeks of gestation, singleton live fetus, with small amount of amniotic fluid. The patient was first treated conservatively with multivitamins and hydration for two weeks before they came to the CiptoMangunkusumo Hospital. In our hospital, the patient and husband were educated regarding the poor prognosis associated with PPROM below 20 weeks and were advised to terminate the pregnancy. It was then decided to terminate the pregnancy. It was the first pregnancy for the patient, and it was expected to be the first grandchild for both parents of the patient. After delivery, both the patient and husband had a difficult time coping. PPROM impacts the biopsychosocial aspects of both maternal and neonates. Mothers might be at risk for systemic infection even after delivery, while newborn babies might be at high risk of respiratory distress syndrome, NEC, or prolonged intubation, which leads to stress and financial burden on the parents. The feelings of separation and exclusion with their baby could be related to the lack of physical and emotional closeness, which are essential factors in the early relationship between parents and their newborn infant. Mothers may also experience several and often conflicting emotional reactions, such as grief, sadness, guilt, fear, anger, loss of self-esteem, and sense of failure. Comprehensive education using a multidisciplinary approach is critical to have the best decisions from parents regarding pregnancy condition. PPROM below 20 weeks likely negatively impacts the parent's physical, emotional, and socio-cultural aspects. Therefore, proper comprehensive education using a holistic approach must be given to reduce the negative impacts.

Keywords: PPROM, preterm birth, biopsychosocial, stress

INTRODUCTION

Each year there are 15 million preterm babies born with a variety of survival chances [1] In middle income and countries with an emerging economy, around 3.8 million preterm babies are born each year, and some countries such as Turkey and Sri Lanka have seen a doubling of deaths for preterm babies over the last decade. Over three quarters of the world's newborn deaths are due to preterm birth complications [2]. Preterm birth has become the second highest cause of death for infants following infection, and has become one of the main causes of death during the first month of life, contributing up to 35% of all neonatal deaths annually [3, 4].

According to the WHO, preterm birth is defined as all babies born earlier than 37 weeks. 80% of premature babies are born between 32 and 37 weeks of gestation, and 5% are born before 28 weeks gestation. At this age, intensive care would be needed to save most of these infants [5]. In 1990, babies born before 25 weeks survived although the latter have a higher risk of impairment. Preterm premature rupture of membranes (PPROM) represents one-third of preterm deliveries. Rupture of membranes before 24 weeks impacted 0.4% of pregnancies and carried a mortality rate of 70% in 2000. Considering this information, termination of pregnancy becomes immediate management in cases of very early rupture of membranes [6]. In addition, the most common impairments are respiratory distress syndrome (RDS), necrotizing enterocolitis, and intraventricular hemorrhage (IVH). Also, long term complications such as neurological impairment (i.e., cerebral palsy, mental retardation, schizophrenia) can also occur [7-13]. Impairment outcomes place a heavy financial and psychological burden on families and the health system [14].

This was the patient's first pregnancy after getting married, and the child was going to be the first grandchild for her parents. The patient's mother is a nurse in the neurology department at RSCM, and the patients live in their parent's house along with four other family members. The patient is a housewife and graduated from high school. The husband is an industrial worker with monthly income IDR 4,000,000/month. Currently, the patient and family are having a difficult time coping with the loss of their child and are cautious about pursuing another pregnancy.

Case Illustration

A 25-year-old female came to the CiptoMangunkusumo hospital due to PPROM for 2 weeks. At that time the patient was diagnosed with PPROM they were in G1 and 17 weeks pregnant with a single intrauterine live fetus and hydramnios. At first, the patient went to an obstetric clinic, and since there was no sign of intrauterine infection, the patient was advised to consume medication and hydrate with at least five liters per day for two weeks. However, one week after treatment, the patient went back to the clinic, and it was determined that there was a small change in amniotic fluid. Therefore, the patient came directly to the CiptoMangunkusumo Hospital for further treatment.

At the CiptoMangunkusumo hospital, the patient was diagnosed with PPROM at 14 days on Gravida 1 19 WGA; singleton lives intrauterine with severe oligohydramnios. The pregnancy was terminated after considering perinatology advice regarding survival rate, and fetomaternal advice regarding the likely poor prognosis.

DISCUSSION

Preterm birth impacts biological, physiological psychological and social aspects. In this case, PPROM may cause infection on both fetal and maternal that can lead to maternal morbidity. The clinical chorioamnionitis rate is 30%, and the most frequent pathogen detected in amniotic fluid is *Ureaplasmaurealyticum.* This can produce an inflammatory response in both the maternal and fetal membranes. Hocq [15] has a reported presence of E.Coli and sepsis in mothers with a history of PPROM < 25 weeks and latency > 14 days. One patient has undergone laparoscopy with the draining of an abscess and received intravenous therapy due to an E. Coli tubo-ovarian abscess requiring a prolonged hospital stay. The neonatal outcome for PPROM is <20 weeks and a longer duration of endotracheal ventilation ($p = 0.01$), acidic arterial blood gas analysis ($p = 0.05$), 5^{the} minute Apgar score <7 ($p < 0.01$), use of inotropic agent during intensive cardiac monitoring ($p < 0.01$) are required. In addition, other long term complications such as Necrotizing Enterocolitis and limb contractions should be considered 15-17].Considering CiptoMangunkusumo hospital perinatology [18] can treat <25 weeks is 0%, and also the risk of maternal morbidity and poor neonatal outcomes then termination of pregnancy is the right decision taken at that time.

Psychological impacts might affect both baby and parents. Parents will most likely feel helpless regarding the care of their baby (intubation, infusion lines, and feeding tube). However, major stress experienced by parents is related to the separation from their baby and to the loss of their parental role as they had previously imagined it [19]. As suggested by Flacking et al. [20], the feelings of separation and exclusion could be related to the lack of physical and emotional closeness, which are important factors in the early relationship between parents and the newborn infant. As frequently reported in the literature, the first moments of the postpartum period are fundamental for the construction of early parent-infant bonding [21]. During hospitalization of their baby, mothers may experience several and often contradictory emotional reactions, such as grief, sadness, guilt, fear, anger, loss of self-esteem, and sense of failure.

Despite the physiological effect, parents might run into financial problems due to prolonged intensive care for early preterm babies [14, 22]. In the USA, medical costs on infants with a birth weight of 500 to 999 grams, cost an estimated $67,0727 to $221,450. Another cost associated with preterm babies are post-discharge parental out-of-pocket expenses and lost productivity [23].

Tommiska et al. [24] documented the first year parental wage losses at around €5,990 for infants with birth weights of <1,000 grams whereas the loss was only €880 for controls. It is predicted that the cost will be higher when babies are born at 20 weeks.

Preterm birth may cause post-traumatic stress disorder (PTSD) due to complications related to maternal and neonatal outcomes. Therefore this condition can trigger negative thoughts regarding their child's appearance and behavior [19, 21, 25]. In fact, this situation can be so overwhelming for mothers that they might react by emotionally distancing themselves from their children [26].

To avoid these negative impacts, psychological (emotional) support must be given at first antenatal care. This support can be given not only from the obstetricians but also other health workers, peer groups and close family members itself [22]. If signs of depression are detected, then additional treatment from a psychiatric professional may be required [27, 28]. As obstetricians, we have to detect any potential problems (biological, psychological, social, and cultural) in every patients, so that we can educate patients in advance. Socio-cultural support can be given by close family members and through religion groups. Though it is considered a small aspect in daily practice, socio-cultural aspects may require the individual to decline our education to parents regarding their baby care [29].

Thus, to provide comprehensive counseling, as an obstetrician, we need a holistic and multidisciplinary approach. In this case, counseling must be given not only from obstetricians but also neonatologist to parents and close family members. After understanding the counseling, we hope that parents can make the best decisions regarding their pregnancy. In this case, termination of the pregnancy has been considered as a best decision taken at that time based on the bio-psychosocial aspects.

Conclusion

PPROM below 20 weeks might cause long-term complication that requires prolonged intensive care. This situation might cause negative physical, emotional and socio-cultural impacts on parents. Therefore, proper comprehensive education using a holistic approach must be given to avoid negative impacts.

References

[1] Blencowe, H., Cousens, S., Oestergaard, M., Chou, D., Moller, A., Narwal, R., Adler, A., Vera Garcia., C., Rohde, S., Say, L. and Lawn, J. E. (2012). National, regional, and worldwide estimates of preterm birth rates in the year 2010 with time trends since 1990 for selected countries: a systematic analysis and implications. *Lancet,* 379: 2162-2172.

[2] Lawn, J., Kinney, M., Belizan, J., Mason, E., McDougall, L., Larson, J., Lackritz, E., Friberg, I. K. and Christopher P Howson, the Born Too Soon Preterm Birth Action Group. (2013). Born Too Soon:

Accelerating action for preventions and care of 15 million newborns born too soon. *Reproductive Health,* 10(Suppl 1):S6.

[3] Liu, L., Johnson, H. L, Cousens, S., Perin, J., Scott, S., Lawn, J. E, Rudan, I., Campbell, H., Cibulskis, R., Li, M., Mathers, C., Black, R. E. and Child Health Epidemiology Reference Group of WHO and UNICEF. (2012). Global, regional, and national causes of child mortality: an updated systematic analysis for 2010 with time trends since 2000. *The Lancet,* 379(9832): 2151-2161.

[4] Lawn, J., Cousens, S. and Zupan, J. (2005). 4 million neonatal deaths: when? Where? Why? *Lancet,* 365(9462): 891-900.

[5] Blencowe, H., Cousens, S., Chou, D., Oestergaard, M., Say, L., Moller, A. B, Kinney, M., Lawn, J. and Born Too Soon Preterm Birth Action Group. (2013). Born Too Soon: The global epidemiology of 15 million preterm births. *Reproductive Health,* 10(Suppl 1):S3.

[6] Williams, O., Hutchings, G., Debiève, F. and Debauche, C. (2009). Contemporary neonatal outcome following rupture of membranes prior to 25 weeks with prolonged oligohydramnios. *Early Human Development,* 85(5): 273-277.

[7] Moreira, R. S, Magalhães, L. C, Alves, C. R. L. (2014). Effect of preterm birth on motor development, behavior, and school performance of school-age children: a systematic review. *Jornal de Pediatria,* 90(2): 119-134.

[8] Simhan, H. N., Berghella, V. and Iams, J. D. Preterm labor and birth. In: Creasy RK, Resnik R, Iams JD, Lockwood CJ, Moore T, Greene MF, editors. (2013). *Creasy and Resnik'smaternal-fetal medicine: principles and practice: expert consult premium edition- enhanced online features.* Elsevier Health Sciences: 624-53.

[9] Marlow, N. (2004). Outcome following extremely preterm birth. *Current Paediatrics*, 14(4): 275-283.

[10] Marlow, N. and Johnson, S. (2012). Outcome following preterm birth. In: Rennie JM, editor. *Rennie & Roberton's Textbook of Neonatology.* 5 ed. London: Elsevier Health Sciences UK: 71-88.

[11] Platt, M. J. (2014). Outcomes in preterm infants. *Public Health,* 128(5): 399-403.

[12] Berbis, J., Einaudi, M. A., Simeoni, M. C., Brevaut-Malaty, V., Auquier, P., d'Ercole, C. and Gire, C. (2012). Quality of life of early school-age French children born preterm: a cohort study. *European Journal of Obstetrics & Gynecology and Reproductive Biology,* 162(1): 38-44.

[13] Roberts, G., Burnett, A. C., Lee, K. J., Cheong, J., Wood, S. J., Anderson, P. J, Doyle, L. W. and Victorian Infant Collaborative Study Group. (2013). Quality of life at age 18 years after extremely preterm birth in the post-surfactant era. *The Journal of Pediatrics,* 163(4): 1008-1013.

[14] Lawn, J. E., Davidge, R., Paul, V. K., Xylander, S. V, Johnson, J. d. G, Costello, A., Kinney, M. V., Segre, Joel. And Molyneux, Liz. (2013). Born too soon: care for the preterm baby. *Reproductive Health,* 10(Suppl 1): S5.

[15] Hocq, C., Grambezen, B. V., Bernard, P. and Debauche, C. (2017). Impact of gestational age at PPROM on the short-term outcome of children born after extreme and prolonged preterm prelabor rupture of membranes in an experienced care center. *SignaVitae,* 13(2): 63-70.

[16] Sungkar, A. and Tanamas, G. (2018). *Karakteristik Kehamilan Terhadap Morbiditas dan Mortalitas Neonatus Pada Kasus Ketuban Pecah Dini Preterm Di Rumah Sakit Cipto Mangunkusumo* [*Pregancy characteristics of neonatal morbidity and mortality in preterm premature rupture of membranes in Dr. Cipto Mangunkusumo Hospital*]. Thesis not yet published.

[17] Verspyck, E., Bisson, V., Roman, H. and Marret, S. (2014). Adverse respiratory outcome after premature rupture of membranes before viability. *Acta Paediatrica,* 103(3): 256-261.

[18] RSCM. (2017). P. *Survival rates of preterm infant in Cipto Mangunkusumo General Hospital.*

[19] Ionio, C., Colombo, C., Brazzoduro, V., Mascheroni, E., Confalonieri, E., Castoldi, F., Listab G. (2016). Mothers and fathers in NICU: the impact of preterm birth on parental distress. *Europe's Journal of Psychology,* 12(4): 604-621.

[20] Flacking, R., Lehtonen, L., Thomson, G., Axelin, A., Ahlqvist, S., Moran, V., Ewald, U., Dykes, F. and Separation and Closeness Experiences in the Neonatal Environment (SCENE) group. (2012). Closeness and separation in neonatal intensive care. *Acta Paediatrica,* 101(10):1032-1037.

[21] Flanagan, J., Maka, E. and Nitulescu, C. (2017). Involving the parents of preterm babies. *Community Eye Health,* 30(99): 60-61.

[22] Lakshmanan, A., Agni, M., Lieu, T., Fleegler, E., Kipke, M., Friedlich, P. S., McCormick, M. C. and Belfort, M. B. (2017). The impact of preterm birth <37 weeks on parents and families: a cross-sectional study in the 2 years after discharge from the neonatal intensive care unit. *Health and Quality of Life Outcomes,* 15(1):38.

[23] Zupancic, J. A. F. A systematic review of costs associated with preterm birth. Behrman R. E., Butler A. S., editors. (2007). Preterm Birth: causes, consequences and prevention. *National Academies Press*: 688.

[24] Tommiska, V., Tuominen, R. and Fellman, V. (2003). Economic costs of care in extremely low birthweight infants during the first 2 years of life. *Pediatric Critical Care Medicine,* 4(2):157-163.

[25] Claire, A., Doornbos, B., Wessel, I. and Aarnouds, J. G. (2011). Postraumatic stress disorder following preeclampsia and PPROM. *Reproductive Sciences,* 18(7): 645-653.

[26] Shah, P., Clements, M. and Poehlmann, J. 2011. Maternal resolution of grief after preterm birth: implications for infant attachment security. *Pediatrics,* 17:284-292.

[27] Jenewein, J., Moergeli, H., Fauchère, J. C., Bucher, H. U., Kraemer, B., Wittmann, L., Schnyder, U. and Büchi, S. 2008. Parents' mental health after the birth of an extremely preterm child: a comparison between bereaved and non-bereaved parents. *Journal of Psychosomatic Obstetrics & Gynecology,* 29(1):53-60.

[28] Schappin, R., Wijnroks, L., UnikenVenema M. M. A. T. And Jongmans, M. J. 2013. Rethinking stress in parents of preterm infants: ameta-analysis. *PLOS One,* 2(2):e54992.

[29] Kucuk, A. D., Kardas, O. F. and Guducu, T. F. 2018. The effect of spiritual care on stress levels of mothers in NICU. *Western journal of nursing research,* 40(7):997-1011.

In: Obstetric and Gynecology Case Report ISBN: 978-1-53616-711-5
Editor: Dwiana Ocviyanti

Chapter 3

UNINTENDED PREGNANCY IN UNMARRIED WOMEN IN INDONESIA

Imam Rahmadi[1,*] and Dwiana Ocviyanti[2]

[1]Faculty of Medicine, Universitas Indonesia, Jakarta, Indonesia

[2]Department of Obstetric and Gynecology, Faculty of Medicine, Universitas Indonesia, Dr. Cipto Mangunkusumo Hospital, Jakarta, Indonesia

ABSTRACT

Pregnancy among unmarried women is far more likely to be unintended and have negative effects. Women who carry unintended pregnancies are more likely to experience pregnancy-related problems, delayed antenatal care, adverse birth outcomes, such as preterm birth and low birth weight, and adverse socioeconomic consequences, such as psychosocial stress and poor mental health. A 30-year-old woman presented at Dr. Cipto Mangunkusumo Hospital with premature rupture of amniotic membranes at 39 weeks of gestation. She had undergone a caesarian section. Both this pregnancy and her previous one were

* Corresponding Author's E-mail: imam2krahmadi@gmail.com.

unintended, and she was unmarried during both. She had not received ANC at any public or private health services. The patient was a freelance worker and resided with her first child. Compared with pregnancies in married women, those among unmarried women tend to occur at a younger age among those with a lower educational level and among those who are unemployed or living in poverty. Women who experience unwanted pregnancies are 2.1 times more likely not to make maximum use of ANC care. Additionally, they are less motivated to seek information regarding the health of their pregnancies. The importance of preventing unintended pregnancies, especially in low economic status communities, can be achieved by health promotion and government prioritization of the screening of women with unintended pregnancies and implementation of the first thousand days of life program from Indonesia Minsitry of Health. Unwanted pregnancies affect ANC behavior. The effect of unwanted pregnancy status varies according to the mother's economic status.

Keywords: unintended pregnancy, unmarried woman, antenatal care

Introduction

The World Health Organization estimates that of the 200 million pregnancies a year. Approximately 75 million are unwanted [1]. This is an important issue that requires attention, especially in developing countries. According to the Indonesian Demographic and Health Survey (IDHA), 2012, 7% of births were unexpected, and 7% were not desired [2].

Case Report

A 30-year-old woman presented at Dr. Cipto Mangunkusumo Hospital with premature rupture of membranes (PROM). She had a history of a caesarian section. She had not received any antenatal care (ANC) at private or public health services, was unsure of the length of her pregnancy, and could not recall the date of her last menstrual period. This was her second unplanned pregnancy out of marriage.

The patient acknowledged that she was in a relationship with a man who has a wife. She chose not to marry or become his second wife. The patient resides in a rented house with her first child, also resulting from an unplanned pregnancy outside marriage. The patient manages several artists, some of whom are not well known. Thus, her monthly income fluctuates; she thus works hard to provide for herself and her child. The patient's boyfriend does not provide any financial support to her or her unborn child.

The patient was diagnosed as multigravida, at 39 weeks of gestational age with a singleton live head presentation, and PROM of 6 hours. No fetal anatomical abnormalities were detected via ultrasound examination. Blood count, urinalysis, urea and creatinine levels were within normal limits. A caesarian section was performed, and a baby boy weighing 4000 g was delivered.

DISCUSSION

Pregnancy among unmarried women is far more likely to be unintended and to have negative effects on both the pregnant woman and her child than among married women [3]. Women who carry unintended pregnancies to a live birth are more likely to experience pregnancy-related problems, delayed prenatal care [4], and adverse socioeconomic consequences, such as psychosocial stress and poor mental health [3].

Compared with married women, pregnancies among unmarried women tend to occur at a younger age, among those with a lower educational level, among the unemployed, and among those in poverty [5]. Other factors associated with pregnancy in unmarried women include the earlier initiation of sexual activity, non-consensual sexual intercourse at first sexual experience, multiple sexual partners, and less use of a condom [6].

Unwanted pregnancies can be caused by unhealthy behavior and conditions at the time before or during pregnancy, such as rape, a lack of contraception knowledge, too many children, health reasons, a disabled fetus, a young age or not ready to have children, irresponsible partners, or unstable relationships with partners. Furthermore, the incidence of unwanted pregnancy is closely associated with various aspects such as the sociodemographic conditions of the family and the culture and beliefs that exist within the community [2].

Abdallah et al. found that 13.4% of women who had unintended pregnancies were illiterate compared with 4.1% illiteracy in women who had intended pregnancies, and the percentage of women from low-income families who had unwanted pregnancies was 15.9%, compared with 4.1% of women from low-income families who had intended pregnancies [7]. Gipson et al. showed that the risk of having unwanted pregnancies in women under the age of 20 years was 2.7 times and that in women over the age of 35 years was 2.3. Furthermore, unmarried women had a 2.5 times risk of experiencing an unwanted pregnancy rather than an intended pregnancy [8]. The impact of abortion on unwanted pregnancies must also be considered since this also affects the pregnancy process and outcome.

A study conducted by Anggraini using the 2012 IDHS data showed that mothers who had an unwanted pregnancy had the odds of 1.4 for not receiving complete ANC compared with those with desired pregnancy [9]. The results of this study are also similar to those of Humbert et al., which demonstrated that women who experience an unwanted pregnancy are 2.1 times more likely not to make maximum use of ANC [10].

Women with unwanted pregnancies are less motivated to seek information regarding the health of their pregnancies, making them more likely to partake in unhealthy behavior because they do not care about the risks to their unborn child. Previous research has revealed that mothers with unwanted pregnancies use fewer health services, receive inadequate nutrition, and experience stress and depression [11]. Nakku et al. revealed a 13% prevalence of postpartum depression that was influenced by factors such as depression during pregnancy, anxiety regarding taking care of their infant, the everyday pressures of life, the spousal relationship, and the interference of physical disorders in both the mother and her baby [12].

CONCLUSION

The amount of unwanted pregnancies remains high. Unwanted pregnancies can affect the behavior of mothers if they are unable to perform optimally. Antenatal care visits are neglected because mothers with an unwanted pregnancy hope that the pregnancy will not continue. The influence of unwanted pregnancy status on maternal behavior during pregnancy and after birth is also influenced by the mother's economic status. The poor are more likely not to receive Antenatal care and complete basic immunization for their baby. Those who are wealthier tend not to provide exclusive breastfeeding [13]. In our case, the mother had little knowledge of the importance of ANC.

There are several actions that can be implemented to prevent or recognize unintended pregnancy. The importance of preventing unintended pregnancies, especially in low economic status communities, and improving maternal and infant health through health promotion needs to be emphasized. Screening for cases of women with unwanted pregnancy status should be performed with the assistance of health workers. Therefore, health workers can provide education to encourage mothers to make use of maternal and child health programs. Identification of the pregnancy status as intended or unintended should become standard practice when providing health services, and the first thousand days of life program from Indonesian Ministry of Health can be implemented well by every pregnant woman.

REFERENCES

[1] Glasier, A, Gulmezoglu, AM, Schmid, GP, Moreno, CG, Van Look, PF. (2006). Sexual and reproductive health: a matter of life and death. *Lancet,* 368: 1595-1607.

[2] BKKBN. (2008). *Unwanted Pregnancy among Couples of reproductive age in Bali*. Jakarta. *BKKBN*.

[3] Raatikainen, K, Heiskanen, N, Heinonen, S. (2005). Marriage still protects pregnancy. *BJOG,* 112: 1411-1416.

[4] Hohmann-Marriott, B. (2009). The couple context of pregnancy and its effects on prenatal care and birth outcomes. *Matern Child Health J,* 13: 745-754.

[5] Jordal, M, Wijewardena, K, Olsson, P. (2013). Unmarried women's ways of facing single motherhood in Sri Lanka - a qualitative interview study. *BMC Women's Health,* 13:5.

[6] Ma, Q, Ono-Kihara, M, Cong, L, Xu, G, Pan, X, Zamani, S, Ravari, SM, Kihara M. (2008). Unintended pregnancy and its risk factors among university students in Eastern China. *Contraception,* 77: 108-113.

[7] Abdallah, IM, Mone'm, EFA, Hassan, M. (2011). Determinants and outcomes of unintended pregnancy among women in Helwan District. *J Am Sci*, 7: 497-505.

[8] Gipson, JD, Koenig, MA, Hindin, MJ. (2008). The effects of unintended pregnancy on infant, child, and parental health: a review of the literature. *Stud Fam Plann,* 39: 18-38.

[9] Anggraini, K. (2014). Pregnancy and K1 and K4 *Examination Behavior in Reproductive Age Women in Indonesia (2012 IDHS Data Analysis)*. Universitas Indonesia.

[10] Humbert, L, Saywell, RM Jr, Zollinger, TW, Priest, CF, Reger, MK, Kochhar, K. (2011). The effect of pregnancy intention on important maternal behaviors and satisfaction with care in a socially and economically at-risk population. *Matern Child Health J,* 15: 1055-1066.

[11] Dye, TD, Wojtowycz, MA, Aubry, RH, Quade, J, Kilburn, H. (1997). Unintended pregnancy and breast-feeding behavior. *Am J Public Health,* 87: 1709-1711.

[12] Nakku, J, Nakasi, G, Mirembe, F. (2006). Postpartum major depression at six weeks in primary health care: prevalence and associated factors. *Afr Health Sci*, 6: 207-214.

[13] Lisa Indrian Dini, PR, Ning, S. (2016). Effect of Unintended Pregnancy towards Mothers' Behaviour during Prenatal and Postnatal in Indonesia (An Analysis of IDHS 2012). *Repro Health J*, 7:119-33.

In: Obstetric and Gynecology Case Report
Editor: Dwiana Ocviyanti
ISBN: 978-1-53616-711-5

Chapter 4

SAFE AND CLEAN DELIVERY

David Eka Prasetya* and Dwiana Ocviyanti
Department of Obstetric and Gynecology, Faculty of Medicine,
Universitas Indonesia, Dr. Cipto Mangunkusumo Hospital,
Jakarta, Indonesia

ABSTRACT

Reproductive health has attracted special attention since the topic was first araised at the International Conference on Population and Development in Cairo, Egypt, in 1994. At the conference, it was agreed to change the paradigm of managing population problems and development via control of population and fertility to focus on reproductive health and fulfillment of reproductive rights. Article 71 of Law Number 36 of 2009 concerning health states that reproductive health must consider biophysical, mental, and social aspects together and not merely as the condition of being free from disease or disability related to the system, functions, and reproductive process in males and females. We have reported Indonesian demographics regarding pregnant women, labor, and family planning until 2018 [1,2].

* Corresponding Author's Email: oryzagrass@yahoo.com.

Keywords: safe and clean deliveries, RIKESDA, reproductive health, child marriage

INTRODUCTION

Strategic issues of reproductive health that need to be considered in Indonesia currently include strategies to lower maternal and infant mortality rates. In an effort to improve a quality public health degree. A World Health Organization (WHO) report published in March 7, 2013, titled "*Married Adolescents*," stated that the United Nations Population Fund (UNFPA) had estimated that between 2011 and 2020, > 140 million women will had married young (short or long term), which means that 14.2 million girls every year or 39,000 every day married young. Of those 140 million females who will marry before the age of 18 years, 50 million will be < 15 years. A child marriage is a human rights violation that can have adverse effects on the education, health, and long-term prospects of females. According to Babatunde Osotimehin, MD, Executive Director, UNFPA, "A girl who is married as a child is a girl whose potential will not be fulfilled." at that time the level knowledge about pregnancy is very low, which leads to various complications during both pregnancy and childbirth. The maternal and infant mortality rates in Indonesia are the highest among the countries included the Association of Southeast Asian Nations, with annual maternal deaths reaching 450 per 100,000 live births, which is far above the maternal mortality rates in Philippines (170 per 100,000 live births) and Thailand (44 per 100,000 life births) (*Indonesian Health Profile, 2010).*

CASE PRESENTATION

Young married women are more vulnerable to sexual partner violence and sexual abuse than *older* married women, including those who marry at an older age. Complications in pregnancy and childbirth are the main causes of death in young women aged 15–19 years [3,4,5]. Young females who marry later and postpone pregnancy beyond their teenage years have more opportunities to stay healthy, improve their education, and build a better life for themselves and their families [4,5,6,7]. The results of the 2018 RIKESDA showed that the youngest recorded age for a married female was 10 years and the oldest was 54 years and that there were many pregnancies in very poor women reported for K1 coverage (*initial pregnancy visits*), with the lowest recorded pregnancy rate being 63% in Papua province and the highest rate of initial pregnancies of 94.4% in DI Yogyakarta, which also had the highest number of check-ups by midwives (85%). Most (62.7%) birth attendants were midwives. The highest proportion (29%) of childbirths occurred at independent midwife practices and 16% occurred at home with assistance from midwives. [10]

DISCUSSION

Four factors that increase maternal mortality have been identified: too young to give birth (aged < 21 years), too old to give birth (aged > 35 years), too short of an interval between births (< 3 years), and too many children (> 2). The proportion of mothers aged < 20 years and > 35 years who die giving birth is 33% of all maternal deaths; therefore, if a family planning program can be implemented well again, it is likely that 33% of maternal deaths could be prevented through contraception. If safe pregnancies are to be prioritized, knowledge regarding safe and clean delivery is needed, both by helpers, especially midwives, and by mothers who want to give birth [8,9].

According to WHO, having knowledge about clean and safe labor is very important. The principles of safe and clean labor are embodied in 3W: Who is an experienced helper, namely, a health professional, such as a *doctor, midwife, or trained nurse*; Where are places that have the *necessary equipment, drugs,* and *other resources*; and what needs to be considered, such as the use of a *partograph* for monitoring, *active management of third-stage labor, hygienic cord cutting* and *binding*, *resuscitation* if necessary, *essential care for newborns* (warmth, early and exclusive care, breastfeeding, and hygiene), *prevention of transmission of human immunodeficiency virus from the mother to the child*, and increase in the *mother's satisfaction and comfort* [8,9,10].

There are six WHO principles for maternal and infant hygiene: *clean hands, clean the perineum, clean everything that will enter the vagina, clean the perineum surface, clean instruments, and clean instruments used for baby cord care, including those for clamping and cutting* [10].

CONCLUSION

To achieve a uniform understanding of how to provide clean and safe labor at delivery, support from various parties is needed. This support includes legal policies from decision makers (government), good relationships between institutions and the government, provision of appropriate guidance to primary health providers, standardization of labor management, sufficient human resources, and improvement in the competence of doctors, midwives, and health workers in charge of delivery services in regional areas. National policies must be able to prepare infrastructure and provide both Yankes and Nakes for delivery services. Monitoring is to be able to control the development and shortcomings or difficulties faced in the service, which are identified in the RIKESDA report, and innovation or development to be able to improve services for a clean and safe delivery.

REFERENCES

[1] BKKBN. (2017). *Survey Demografi dan Kesehatan Remaja* [Demographic and adolescent health survey]. *National Population and Family Planning Agency.*

[2] Ministry of Health, Republic of Indonesia. *RISKESDAS (Basic Health Research)*, 2018. Jakarta: Ministry of Health, Republic of Indonesia.

[3] Azevedo, W.F., Diniz, M.B., Fonseca, E.S., Azevedo, L.M., Evangelista, C.B. (2015). Complications in adolescent pregnancy: systematic review of the literature. *Einstein*, 13: 618-626.

[4] Hodgkinson, S., Beers, L., Southammakosane, C., Lewin, A. (2014). Addressing the mental health needs of pregnant and parenting adolescents. *Pediatrics*, 133: 114-122.

[5] Patch, L.K. (1990). Adolescent pregnancy: psychosocial issues. *Indiana Med,* 83: 30-33.

[6] Shaw, M., Lawlor, D.A., Najman, J.M. (2006). Teenage children of teenage mothers: Psychological, behavioural and health outcomes from an Australian prospective longitudinal study. *Soc. Sci. Med,* 62 : 2526-2539.

[7] Cook, S.M.C., Cameron, S.T. (2015). Social issues of teenage pregnancy. *Obstet. Gynaecol. Reprod. Med,* 25 : 243-248.

[8] Bhandari TR, Kutty VR, Sarma PS, Dangal G. (2017). Safe delivery care practices in western Nepal: Does women's autonomy influence the utilization of skilled care at birth?. *PLoS One*, 12(8). Doi:10.1371/journal.pone.0182485.

[9] Blencowe H, Cousens S, Mullany LC, et al. (2011). Clean birth and postnatal care practices to reduce neonatal deaths from sepsis and tetanus: a systematic review and Delphi estimation of mortality effect. *BMC Public Health*, 11 (3): S11. Doi:10.1186/1471-2458-11-S3-S11.

[10] World Health Organization. (2018). *Adolescents: health risks and solutions*.

In: Obstetric and Gynecology Case Report ISBN: 978-1-53616-711-5
Editor: Dwiana Ocviyanti

Chapter 5

BIOPSYCHOSOCIAL IMPACTS IN PREGNANCY AMONG VICTIMS OF INCEST

David E. Prasetya[1,*] and Dwiana Ocviyanti[1]
[1]Department of Obstetric and Gynecology, Faculty of Medicine, Universitas Indonesia, Dr. Cipto Mangunkusumo Hospital, Jakarta, Indonesia.

ABSTRACT

Incest, a form of child sexual abuse, is a public health concern that has been commonly neglected and concealed. Factors such as inadequate communication skills to recognize the victim and the social inability to manage reports of suspected child sexual abuse may be responsible for this neglect. Global information may play a primary role in influencing sexual content. Victims' silence, and cultural and societal stigma exacerbate the problem. Pregnancy due to incest results in biopsychosocial impacts, thus creating a burden some global health problem. This paper explores a holistic approach from the biological, psychological, and social aspects of a *34-week teenage pregnancy and intrauterine fetal death case.*In the case illustrated in this paper, an 18-year-old pregnant woman was admitted to

* Corresponding Author's E-mail: oryzagrass@yahoo.com.

Ciptoangunkusumo Hospital. She had suffered preterm labor when 34 weeks pregnant, which resulted in intrauterine fetal death. During the pregnancy, it was discovered that she had a history of forced sexual intercouse with her stepfather until she became pregnant. Her mother was too afraid to report it at first, but as her daughter's pregnancy progressed, the mother reported the matter and the father was eventually arrested. According to previous literature, family incest is rarely reported. Generally, children are the victims of rape; in particular, the perpetrators of this sexual violence are fathers and the victims, their daughters. Psychologically, sexual violence or rape destroys the mentality of the victim. Incest is rarely reported to the authorities because of the fear of tarnishing the family name and having a criminal record.

Keywords: family incest, impact incest pregnancy

CASE ILLUSTRATION

The patient was an 18-year-old Sundanese, Muslim G1P0 woman who was unmarried and had dropped out of third grade in high school in Jakarta because she was pregnant. The patient lived with her parents, one of whom was her stepfather as her biological father had died when she was still a baby. She had a 12-year-old stepbrother. Her stepfather was jobless and a drug user; her mother sold *yakult,* a health drink, for a living. The patient discovered she was pregnant at 19 weeks. At first, she would not reveal the father of her child, but at her mother's insistence, she relayed the truth. When the patient's mother confronted her husband, he acted violently toward her. When the patient was six months pregnant, her mother reported the matter to the police and her husband was imprisoned. Thereafter, the mother supported the patient. However, a medical examination revealed the patient was losing amniotic fluid. At 34 weeks, the patient's amniotic fluid was abnormally low despite the fact her water had not broken. Twelve hours before being admitted to Ciptomangunkusumo Hospital the patient was diagnosed with active phase labor at Bayangkara Hospital and referred to Ciptomangunkusumo Hospital. The baby, a 2200 gram baby girl, was delivered preterm at 34 weeks, but died. The patient was taken care of by psychiatric and medico-legal forensic specialists.

Discussion

Every country has its own laws to deal with incest. From a medico-legal aspect, the patient's mother did the right thing because incest is regarded as sexual child assault. In Indonesian law, the father could be charged with violating the following child protection laws: 76D, 287, and/or 294. Furthermore, he could be imprisoned for a maximum of nine years. Many internal factors are involved in incest such as perpetrators' abundance of sexual drive and inability to control their sexual desires (Testoni et al. 2018). This biological factor is difficult to cure. The perpetrator usually being sexually dissatisfied with their wives and loneliness can explain their incestuous relations. Girls in some contries also tend to have a habit of sleeping with their fathers. Furthermore, alleged sexual disorders and psychiatric disorders are often the cause (Collins, Griffiths and Kumalo 2005). Sometimes,to ensure continuity of the bloodline and to ensure that descendants inherit property, royals tend to have incestuous relations (Sheinberg and Fraenkel 2001).

External factors include economic factors and lack of knowledge, especially regarding sex, and religion. Currently, owing to globalization and technological developments, social changes are occurring rapidly. Communication devices such as radio, television, videos, mobile phones, newspapers, and magazines have infiltrated Indonesia. Furthermore, new cultures, contrary to the local culture and norms, can be found in the country. People have easy access to the news about sexual crimes through television shows and articles in newspapers and magazines. They are also able to obtain information about and experience pornography through various forms of media (Stroebel et al. 2012).

Another factor involves the age of the victims who are usually young, have limited resilience, and are afraid of authority figures. This is often evident when a father has an incestuous relationship with his daughter. Often the child does not understand sex. However, the child is often scared of what will happen if she does not succumb to the will of her father. It has been acknowledged that superior authority and fear of adults usually encourage children to do what they are asked to do (Courtois 2010).

Besides sexual violence, victims may suffer many psychological consequences, such as sexual abuse trauma; an inability to trust others; fear or worry in sexual relations; depression, suicide, and other self-destructive behavior; low self-esteem; feelings of guilt; anger; loneliness; an inability to get along with other people; and irregular eating habits. Furthermore, the victim may not care about her pregnancy and suffer from postpartum depression. Moreover, incest can cause damage to the victim's reproductive organs, as they are not fully developed. The victim may also be at risk of contracting sexually transmitted diseases. Victims and offenders suffer stress, which may have a detrimental effect on their mental health. Another impact of incest is the possibility of giving birth to an abnormal child who may have homozigot genes if the biological father is a close relative. Diseases passed down through homozygous recessive genes include fatal anemia, impaired vision or blindness, polydactyl, and albinism. The infant may also die. Incest in a family may result in social conseqences such as family shame in the public's eyes. The family may become isolated from the community and the subject of discussion in the community (Collins et al. 2005). It is also problematic when a child is born because of incest, as the perpetrator is not only related to that child as its father but also as its grandfather.

CONCLUSION

Incest, a form of child sexual abuse, is a public health problem, which is often neglected and concealed. The victims' silence exacerbates the problem, especially in patriarchal communities and in various cultures. Victims suffer biopsychosocial consequences from this global problem. Parents are advised to report incest. Furthermore, victims should be cared for comprehensively and holistically.

REFERENCES

Bauer, A. M., Quas, J. A., Boyce, W. T. (2002). Associations between physiological reactivity and children's behavior: Advantages of a multisystem approach. *Journal of Developmental and Behavioral Pediatrics,* 23:102 - 113.

Collins, S., Griffiths, S. and Kumalo, M. (2005). Patterns of disclosure in child sexual abuse. *South African Journal of Psychology, 35*: 270 - 285. Doi: 10.1177/008124630503500207.

Courtois, C. A. (2010). *Healing the incest wound: Adult survivors in therapy* (2nd ed.). New York, NY: WW Norton & Company.

Ferrara, F. F. (2002). *Childhood sexual abuse: developmental effects across the lifespan.* Australia: Brooks/Cole Thomson Learning.

Kellya, Robert J., Jeffrey J. Wooda, Lauren S. Gonzaleza, Virginia MacDonalda Jill Watermana. (2002). Effects of mother-son incest and positive perceptions of sexual abuse experiences on the psychosocial adjustment of clinic-referred men. *Science Direct.* Doi.org: 10.1016/S0145-2134(02)00317-4.

Kim, K., Noll, J. G., Putnam, F. W., Trickett, P. K. (2007). Psychosocial characteristics of nonoffending mothers of sexually abused girls: Findings from a prospective, multigenerational study. *Child Maltreatment,* 12: 338 - 351.

Owens, G. P. And Chard, K. M. (2003). Comorbidity and psychiatric diagnoses among women reporting child sexual abuse. *Child Abuse and Neglect,* 27 (9):1075 - 1082.

Sheinberg, M., and Fraenkel, P. (2001). *The relational trauma of incest: A family-based approach to treatment*. Guilford Press.

Soron, T. R. (2016). A case report on management of father daughter incest with schizophrenia. *Case Reports in Psychiatry, 3*. doi:10.1155/2016/4010187.

Stroebel, S. S., O'Keefe, S. L., Beard, K. W., Kuo, S. Y., Swindell, S. V., and Kommor, M. J. (2012). Father–daughter incest: Data from an anonymous computerized survey. *Journal of Child Sexual Abuse, 21*(2): 176 - 199. doi:10.1080/10538712.2012.654007.

Testoni, I., Mariani, C. and Zamperini, A. (2018). Domestic violence between childhood incest and re-victimization: A study among anti-violence centers in italy. *Frontiers in Psychology, 9*(2377). doi:10.3389/fpsyg.2018.02377.

Zasmani, S. (2003). *Konseling melalui perspektif Islam: Sumbang mahram* [Counselling through Islamic perspective: Incest]. Proceeding of National Counselling Conference on Islamic Perspective: 81 - 93.

In: Obstetric and Gynecology Case Report ISBN: 978-1-53616-711-5
Editor: Dwiana Ocviyanti

Chapter 6

HOLISTIC AND MULTIDISCIPLINARY APPROACHES IN A GRANDEMULTIPAROUS WOMAN WITH TUBERCULOSIS

Junita Indarti*

Department of Obstetric and Gynecology, Faculty of Medicine, Universitas Indonesia, Dr. Cipto Mangunkusumo Hospital, Jakarta, Indonesia

ABSTRACT

Prevalence of tuberculosis in pregnancy is highly worldwide with more than 200,000 women with active tuberculosis in 2011, especially in Africa and South East Asia. Tuberculosis infection is caused by inhaled *M. tuberculosis* which gets into an active or dormant state. Adequate antenatal care is very important. Our research involved a newborn baby who has a mother with active tuberculosis, and both of them were treated. Mrs A, a 37 year old grandemultiparous woman, exhibited signs of premature labor at 34 weeks' gestation. Upon presentation, she also developed cough,

* Corresponding Author's Email: junita_indarti@yahoo.com.

weight loss, and night sweats. Her chest X-ray showed a bilateral infiltrate pattern, suggestive of tuberculosis. She had a normal delivery at term pregnancy, giving birth to a small baby who was roomed-in with the mother. After being diagnosed with tuberculosis based on clinical and chest X-ray examination, she received a one-month treatment for tuberculosis and was planned to receive a total of six months of treatment. The baby also got isoniazid prophylaxis (INH) therapy for 6 months. Tuberculosis infection in the baby was ruled out, and the baby should be given isoniazid preventive therapy instead, followed by BCG vaccination after 2 weeks of treatment and negative skin test. Management of tuberculosis during pregnancy must be carried out by adopting not only a biological approach but also a psychosocial approach. The management should be disseminated among medical professionals, public health care officials, government agencies, and the patients.

Keywords: holistic approach, multidisciplinary approach, tuberculosis in pregnancy

INTRODUCTION

Prevalence of tuberculosis in pregnancy is highly worldwide with more than 200,000 pregnant women with active tuberculosis in 2011, especially in Africa and South East Asia. In the United States, from 2003 to 2011, the number of incidence of tuberculosis in pregnancy was 26.6 per 100,000 births. Tuberculosis infection is caused by inhaled *M. tuberculosis* which gets into an active or dormant state. Adequate antenatal care is important for pregnant women who are suspected and diagnosed with tuberculosis. The aim of antenatal care is to treat active and latent tuberculosis, especially for patients with low compliance [1, 2].

Patients with latent infection do not show any symptoms, and the disease is not contagious, but the pathogens continue to live and can be reactivated. Activation could be triggered by conditions, such as HIV, diabetes mellitus, and the pregnancy itself. Tuberculosis screening is suggested if there is clinical suspicion manifesting in risk factors, such as travelling to an endemic place [1, 2].

A mother with active tuberculosis must be isolated from her baby, and then evaluation should be performed. If both mother and baby suffer from active tuberculosis, both of them are treated. The mother can nurture her baby, but she should use a mask. If Mantoux test result is negative, the baby should be treated as having latent tuberculosis for 3 months. BCG vaccine cannot be given during pregnancy, because it is a live vaccine. During lactation, for latent tuberculosis anti-tuberculosis drug is still given. Active tuberculosis is treated 2 weeks prior to lactation [1, 2].

We present a case of a mother and her newborn baby who were both treated for tuberculosis because the mother had an active tuberculosis infection. The mother discontinued breastfeeding 3 weeks postpartum and was educated to re-lactate.

Case Report

A 37-year-old grandemultiparous married woman exhibited signs of premature labor at 34 weeks' gestation. She had also developed a cough, weight loss, and night sweats, but there was no history of hemoptysis during the pregnancy period. She denied any contact with tuberculosis and had not previously received a BCG vaccination. She was a housewife with six children, the eldest being 16 years old and the youngest 16 months old.

Results of physical examination in the form of chest auscultation revealed diffuse faint crepitations throughout both lung fields. Her chest X-ray showed a bilateral infiltrate pattern, suggestive of tuberculosis. She was hospitalized and received tocolytics and steroids to promote lung maturation due to threatened preterm labor. Sputum was not collected for analysis. Her pregnancy continued to term. Following a normal delivery, she gave birth to a small baby who was roomed-in with her. She underwent post-placental insertion of an intrauterine contraceptive device. Due to her circumstances (i.e., her husband was in Oman, she had to take care of her six other children, and she had to attend college every day), she did not feel confident to breastfeed her baby. She attempted to breastfeed during the first day after her baby's birth, but her quantity of milk was insufficient, making her even more uncertain about breastfeeding. She discontinued breastfeeding at 3 weeks postpartum. We educated her to attempt to re-lactate her baby. She received sufficient medication for 1 month of a planned 6-month treatment for tuberculosis. The baby received isoniazid prophylactic (INH) therapy for 6 months. The mother's other children had not yet been screened for tuberculosis.

Discussion

Findings and Diagnosis of Tuberculosis

Tuberculosis can be identified through physical and laboratory examinations, resulting in early detection, diagnosis, and severity classification of the disease. Detection can be either active or passive, involving screening at-risk populations (such as HIV patients, prisoners, low socioeconomic populations, infants living with an active tuberculosis patient, and people who have contacted with drug-resistant tuberculosis) and health promotion among the general public [3].

Tuberculosis diagnosis is made by physical examinations, radiologic investigations, and laboratory tests on pregnant and non-pregnant women. The main symptom of tuberculosis is cough which lasts for more than 2 to 3 weeks, and this could be complicated with hemoptysis, dyspnea, malaise, poor appetite, night sweats without any physical activity, and fever which lasts for more than 1 month. However, other diseases, such as bronchiectasis, chronic bronchitis, asthma, and lung cancer, also exhibit similar symptoms. Thus, laboratory examination of a series of three sputum specimens is required to screen for the presence of *M. tuberculosis*. The tuberculin test and interferon gamma release assay are also recommended for tuberculosis screening and diagnosis [3, 4]. The procedures for tuberculosis screening and diagnosis for pregnant women include the tuberculin sensitivity test followed by the sputum test and chest X-ray. Tuberculin test and IGRA are recommended for tuberculosis screening and diagnosis [3, 4].

Table 1. Edward's score for tuberculosis diagnosis in pediatric patients. A total score of >7 is indicative of tuberculosis

Feature/score	0	1	2	3
Edwards' Score [11, 12]				
Duration of illness (in weeks)	<2	2-4		>4
Nutrition (% weight for age)	>80	60-80		<60
Family history of tuberculosis	None	Reported by family		Proven sputum positive
Tuberculin test				Positive
Malnutrition				Not improving after 4 weeks
Unexplained fever				
New modified Edwards' score	Pathozyme tuberculosis complex test			
Duration of illness (in weeks)	<2	2-4		
Nutrition (% weight for length)	>80	60-80		
Family history of tuberculosis	None	Reported by family		Proven sputum positive
Tuberculin test				Positive
Malnutrition				Not improving after 4 weeks
Unexplained fever (>2 weeks)			No response to treatment	

For infants born from mothers with an active disease, tuberculosis drug is given, and the condition is treated like latent tuberculosis for 6 months. After 6 months, the tuberculin skin test is performed; if the skin test is negative, BCG vaccine is given (Table 1) [5].

Treatment

Tuberculosis treatment is given to cure the patient, prevent death, prevent relapse of tuberculosis infections, break the chain of spread, and prevent the development of drug-resistant tuberculosis strains. A single-drug treatment is never given, and a fixed-dose combination is recommended (Table 2) [3].

Table 2. List of anti-tuberculosis drugs

Drug	Recommended dose			
	Daily		3 times per week	
	Dose and range (mg/kg body weight)	Maximum (mg)	Dose and range (mg/kg body weight)	Daily Maximum (mg)
Isoniazid	5 (4-6)	300	10 (8-12)	900
Rifampicin	10 (8-12)	600	10 (8-12)	600
Pyrazinamide	25 (20-30)	-	35 (30-40)	-
Ethambutol	15 (15-20)	-	30 (25-35)	-
Streptomycin*	15 (12-18)		15 (12-18)	1000

* Patients aged over 60 years may not be able to tolerate more than 500-750 mg daily, so some guidelines recommend reduction of the dose to 10 mg/kg per day in patients belonging to this age group (2). Patients weighing less than 50 kg may not tolerate doses above 500-750 mg daily (*WHO Model Formulary 2008*, www.who.int/selection_medicine/list/en/).

Tuberculosis drugs are given in two phases: intensive and continuation phases. The intensive phase occurs during the first 2 months of treatment, while the continuation phase gives fewer drugs in a longer period, aimed at ensuring that all persistent bacteria are eliminated to prevent relapse. The same guidelines apply to pregnant women with prior education and counseling [3, 4].

The first line drugs used for pregnant women include isoniazid (INH), ethambutol (ETB), and rifampicin (RIF). In infants whose mothers have an active tuberculosis infection, tuberculosis drugs are given to the mothers, while the infants are treated as having latent tuberculosis for 6 months. Thereafter, a tuberculin skin test is performed. If the baby's skin test is negative, a BCG vaccine is given [5].

Tuberculosis demands a long term treatment which needs good compliance and persistent availability of drugs. In pregnant women, the treatment course is similar to that of normal patients. All tuberculosis drugs are safe, except streptomycin. Rifampicin could interact with hormonal contraception and could reduce the effectiveness of hormonal contraception. Non-hormonal contraception is preferred for tuberculosis patients. Education and counseling for drug side effect should be provided for patients. Continuity of drug administration and prevention of bad compliance could be carried out by a drug supervisor [5].

Breastfeeding for active tuberculosis mothers is allowed, but the mothers should receive full-course tuberculosis treatment. During breastfeeding, mothers must wear a mask to prevent the airborne transmission of the disease. Mother and baby should stay together, and breastfeeding should be continued. Pyridoxine supplementation is recommended for all pregnant or breastfeeding mothers who are taking isoniazid. Anti-tuberculosis drugs are secreted in small amount in breast milk and do not have toxic effect on babies [6, 7].

Contraception Authority

The authority over contraception in Indonesia is specified in the Constitutional Law of the Republic of Indonesia Number 36 of 2009 concerning health (Articles 5, 71, and 78) and the Law of the Republic of Indonesia Number 52 of 2009 concerning population and family development. Contraception is the right of every person, which is equal for both wife and husband. Contraception is applied by mutual consent of both husband and wife after they are given counseling by professional health workers [8, 9]. In our study, the wife (our patient) wanted sterilization contraception, but the husband did not approve. This became a problem because in Indonesian culture, the husband is regarded as the leader in the family, and therefore, based on the correct medical procedures, the husband's consent is needed.

Breastfeeding in Tuberculosis Patients and Re-Lactation

A breastfeeding woman who has tuberculosis should receive a full course of tuberculosis treatment. Timely and properly applied therapy is the best way to prevent transmission of tubercle bacilli to the baby. Mother and baby should stay together and the baby should continue to breastfeed. After active tuberculosis in the baby is ruled out, the baby should be given a 6-month isoniazid preventive therapy, followed by BCG vaccination. Pyridoxine supplementation is recommended for all pregnant or breastfeeding women taking isoniazid [7]. Our patient had already received education by Social Pediatric Department and been instructed to continue breastfeeding. The baby had also been ruled out of congenital tuberculosis and given prophylactic treatment with isoniazid. However, due to her many activities, i.e., she had to take care her other six children, she had to go to college every day, and her husband had to go to Oman, she did not feel confident of breastfeeding her baby. She tried to breastfeed during the first days after her baby's birth, but she did not produce a sufficient amount of breast milk. She felt more unconfident of breastfeeding. Therefore, after 3 weeks postpartum, she no longer breastfed her baby.

We advised her to re-lactate her baby. Re-lactation is re-established breastfeeding by a woman who has stopped breastfeeding a child, either her own child or an adopted infant, either recently or in the past, even without further pregnancy. A woman who has never been pregnant can also establish lactation, and this is called induced lactation [10]. In the past, re-lactation and induced lactation were considered exceptional experiences and were not well researched. However, there are now sufficient reports to show that most women can re-lactate if they are motivated and have adequate information and support. Auerbach and Avery have carried out the most substantial study of this, which is a retrospective study performed in the USA. They used the recall method to study four groups of mothers:

1. 174 women who stopped breastfeeding prematurely;
2. 117 women who re-lactated for a low birth weight infant;
3. 75 who resumed breastfeeding after they or their babies had been hospitalized; and
4. 240 women who breastfed an adopted infant, 83 of whom had never been pregnant, 55 of whom had been pregnant but had never breastfed, and 102 of whom had breastfed a previous infant.

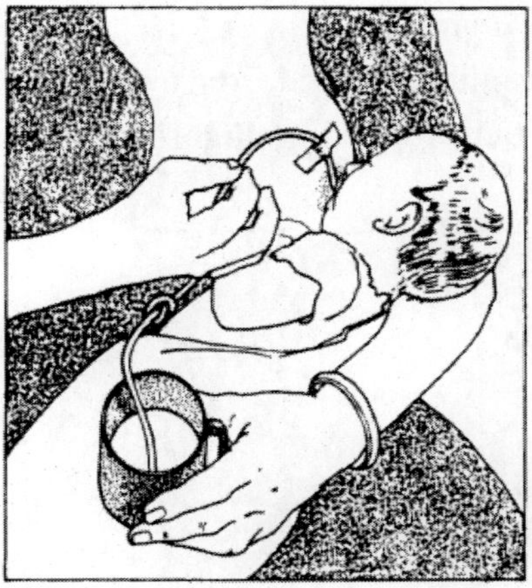

Figure 1. Using a breastfeeding supplement.

There are also a number of reports from developing countries: Papua New Guinea, Nigeria, and India. Re-lactation was successful for all except one of the mothers [10].

Before re-lactation starts, a breastfeeding counselor should talk to the mother. The breastfeeding counselor should ensure that the mother is fully informed about re-lactation and she is adequately motivated. There are some techniques for induced lactation or re-lactation. The important thing is stimulation of the nipple and breast.

If the baby is willing to suckle, encourage the mother to put the baby to her breast frequently, as often as he or she is willing. This should be done once every 1 to 2 hour if possible and at least 8 to 12 times every 24 hours. Let the baby suckle on both breasts as long as possible at each feed, i.e., at least 10 to 15 minutes on each breast. Avoid using a pacifier or bottle. If the baby is unwilling to suckle, the mother could use these techniques [10]:

1. Breastfeeding Supplement

This technique is designed to provide the infant with a steady flow of supplementary feed while he or she suckles and stimulates the breast and nipple. A supplement consists of a bag, bottle, or cup of the milk feed with a fine tube, through which the feed can pass, leading along the nipple to the baby's mouth (Figure 1).

2. Drop and Drip Technique

In this technique, milk is dripped from a dropper or a cup directly onto the breast while the infant is suckling (Figure 2).

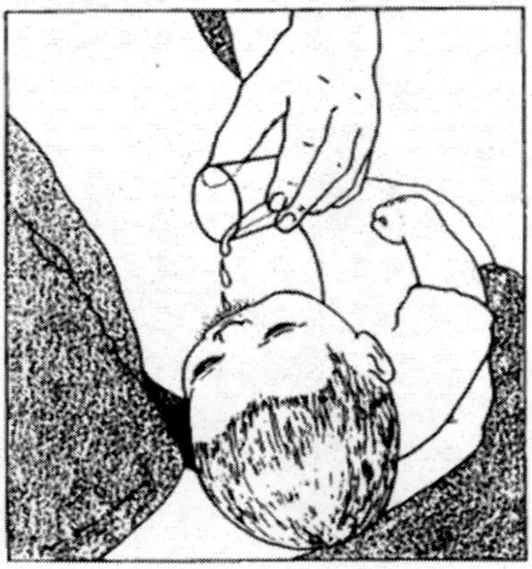

Figure 2. The drop and drip technique.

3. Mechanical and Hand Expression

This technique involves expressing breast milk either manually or mechanically using a hand-operated or electric breast pump (Figure 3).

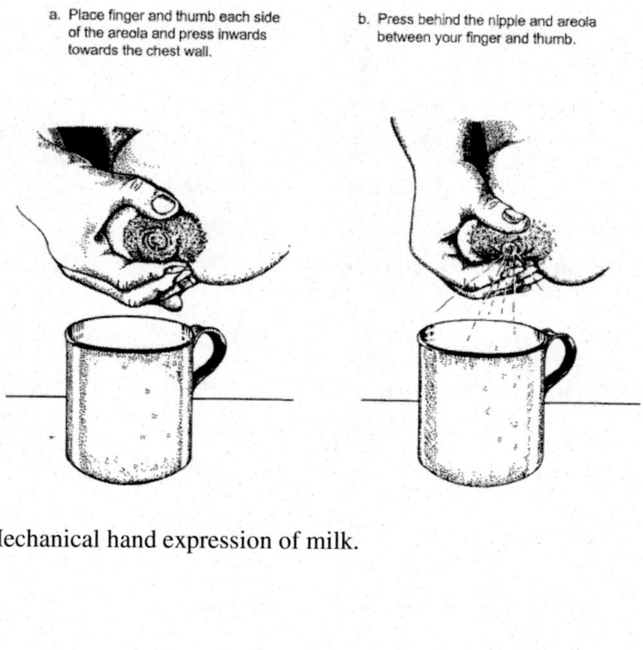
a. Place finger and thumb each side of the areola and press inwards towards the chest wall.
b. Press behind the nipple and areola between your finger and thumb.

Figure 3. Mechanical hand expression of milk.

Table 3. Drugs That Can Be Prescribed to Induce Lactation [11]

Drug	Dosage	Side-effects	Reference	Action
Domperidone	10 mg three times daily	Well tolerated	Petraglia et al., 1985	Blockage of pituitary dopamine receptors
Thyrotrophine-releasing hormone	Nasal spray; 1 mg four times daily	Well tolerated, no clinical signs of hyperthyroidism	Peters et al., 1991	Direct stimulation of adenohypophyseal lactotrophs
Metoclopramide	10 mg three times daily	Well tolerated; fewer side-effects	Banapurmath et al., 1993; Nemba, 1994; Hallbauer, 1997	Blocks dopamine-mediated inhibition of prolactin secretion
Sulpiride	50 mg three times daily	Extrapyramidal symptoms, drowsiness	Hallbauer, 1997	Blocks dopamine-mediated inhibition of prolactin secretion
Chlorpromazine	25-100 mg three times daily	Extrapyramidal symptoms, drowsiness	Brown, 1997; Nema, 1994	Blocks dopamine-mediated inhibition of prolactin secretion

Additionally, there are various drugs that can be administered to induce lactation (Table 3).

Conclusion

The management of tuberculosis during pregnancy should be performed by adopting not only a biological approach but also a psychosocial approach. It should be disseminated among medical professionals, public health care officials, government agencies, and the patients. A biopsychosocial approach by means of education, counseling, identification of social problems encountered by a patient, and detection of a patient's inability to deal with the disease could improve the quality of treatment and could prevent a poor outcome and the spread of the disease from an infected mother to her infant.

REFERENCES

[1] Mathad JS, Gupta A. (2012). Tuberculosis in pregnant and postpartum women: epidemiology, management, and research gaps. *Clin. Infect. Dis*, 55:1532-1549.

[2] Kwan BCH, Yu Y, Goldberg H. (2010). A case of tuberculosis in a pregnant woman and review of current literature. *Obstet. Med*, 3:161-163.

[3] Kementerian Kesehatan RI. (2014). *Pedoman Nasional Pengendalian Tuberkulosis* [*National Guidelines for Tuberculosis Control*]. Jakarta: 6-20.

[4] Harries A, Maher D, Uplekar M, Raviglione M, Chaulet P, Nunn P, Luelmo F, van Praag E. (1997). *TB: A clinical manual for South East Asia.* World Health Organization.

[5] Kimberlin DW, Brady, MT, Jackson, MA editors. (2018). AAP Committee on Infectious Diseases. American Academy of Pediatrics. *Red Book*:1264.

[6] Asik Hastuti EB, Evarini Y. (2016). *Petunjuk teknis manajemen dan tatalaksana TB anak* [*Technical guidelines for management and management of child TB*].Ministry of Health Republic Indonesia:1-81.

[7] World Health Organization. (2010). *Stop TB Dept. Treatment of tuberculosis: guidelines.* 4th ed. Geneva: World Health Organization.

[8] Presiden Republik Indonesia [President of the Republic of Indonesia]. (2009). *Undang-Undang Republik Indonesia No. 36 tahun 2009 tentang Kesehatan* [*Republic of Indonesia Law No. 36 of 2009 concerning Health*] Jakarta.

[9] Presiden Republik Indonesia [President of the Republic of Indonesia]. (2009. *Undang-Undang Republik Indonesia No. 52 tahun 2009 tentang Perkembangan Kependudukan dan Pembangunan Keluarga* [*Republic of Indonesia Law No. 52 of 2009 concerning Population Development and Family Development*] Jakarta.

[10] Hormann E, Savage F. (1998). *Relactation: a review of experience and recommendations for practice.* World Health Organization.

[11] Biervliet FP, Maguiness SD, Hay DM, Killick SR, Atkin SL. (2001). Induction of lactation in the intended mother of a surrogate pregnancy: case report. *Hum. Reprod*, 16:581-583.

In: Obstetric and Gynecology Case Report ISBN: 978-1-53616-711-5
Editor: Dwiana Ocviyanti

Chapter 7

SUCCESSFUL CONSERVATIVE MANAGEMENT OF A HIGH-LEVEL β-hCG CESAREAN PREGNANCY

Herbert Situmorang ***and Duma Margaretha***
Department of Obstetric and Gynecology, Faculty of Medicine, Universitas Indonesia, Dr. Cipto Mangunkusumo Hospital, Jakarta, Indonesia

ABSTRACT

Cesarean scar pregnancy (CSP) is a serious condition in which the embryo implants within the myometrium of a previous cesarean section scar. A standard treatment protocol for this condition has not yet been established as the data remain limited, given the rarity of its occurrence. This case report describes a patient who was diagnosed with a CSP at 12 weeks of gestation with beta-human chorionic gonadotropin (β-hcG) levels of 34,968.12 mIU/mL. She was successfully treated with systemic methotrexate followed by evacuation through a hysteroscopic procedure

* Corresponding Author's Email: dr.duma.margaretha@gmail.com.

using an Integrated Bigatti Shaver. This report adds to the literature on safe and effective treatments for CSP. A 35-year-old, gravida 4, para 3, woman with a history of two prior term cesarean sections was diagnosed with a CSP during a routine first-trimester ultrasound at 12 weeks of gestation. She had reported spotting in the previous 2 weeks. Ultrasound revealed a gestational sac with a diameter of 2.62 cm. Methotrexate 50 mg/m2 was administered as a single dose via intravenous infusion according to the "two-dose regimen," following which β-hcG levels decreased. The present case is an important contribution to the research on CSP treatment. Systemic methotrexate followed by a hysteroscopic procedure is a safe and effective approach for conservative treatment of a first-trimester CSP while preserving fertility.

Keywords: cesarean section scar pregnancy, ectopic pregnancy, methotrexate

INTRODUCTION

Cesarean section scar pregnancy (CSP) is a rare and serious type of ectopic pregnancy in which the embryo implants within the myometrium of a previous cesarean section scar. The condition may lead to serious maternal complications, such as abnormal placentation, hemorrhage, or death due to uterine rupture. Despite these grave consequences, a standard treatment protocol has not yet been established as the data are limited, given the rarity of the occurrence. This case report describes a patient who was diagnosed with a CSP at 12 weeks of gestation. She was successfully treated with systemic methotrexate followed by evacuation through a hysteroscopic procedure using an Integrated Bigatti Shaver (IBS). This report adds to the literature on safe and effective conservative treatments for CSP.

Ectopic pregnancy accounts for approximately 1% of all pregnancies [1, 2]. Furthermore, SCP are rare, only account for 0.05%–0.04% of all pregnancies, and associated with potentially fatal consequences [1, 10-11]. Because the rate of cesarean section has risen in recent years, this type of ectopic pregnancy is relatively rare [3], 40% of the CSP cases being asymptomatic [4]. To preserve maternal fertility, diagnosis and treatment are important. Although termination of preganancy was recommended as soon as possible, definitive theurapeutic approached still remain unclear [5]. The treatment for CSP are consist of medical therapy, (by using methotrexate) and surgical interventions (by using bigatti shaver, as scar wedge resection and hysterectomy) [1, 6]. This case report illustrates the CSP case in the first-trimester by using systemic methotrexate followed by a hysteroscopic procedure helped achieve a successful and safe outcome.

CASE REPORT

A 35-year-old, gravida 4, para 3, woman with a history of two prior term cesarean sections was diagnosed with a CSP during a routine first-trimester ultrasound at 12 weeks of gestation (Figure 1). The ultrasound showed the gestational sac diameter to be 2.62 cm.

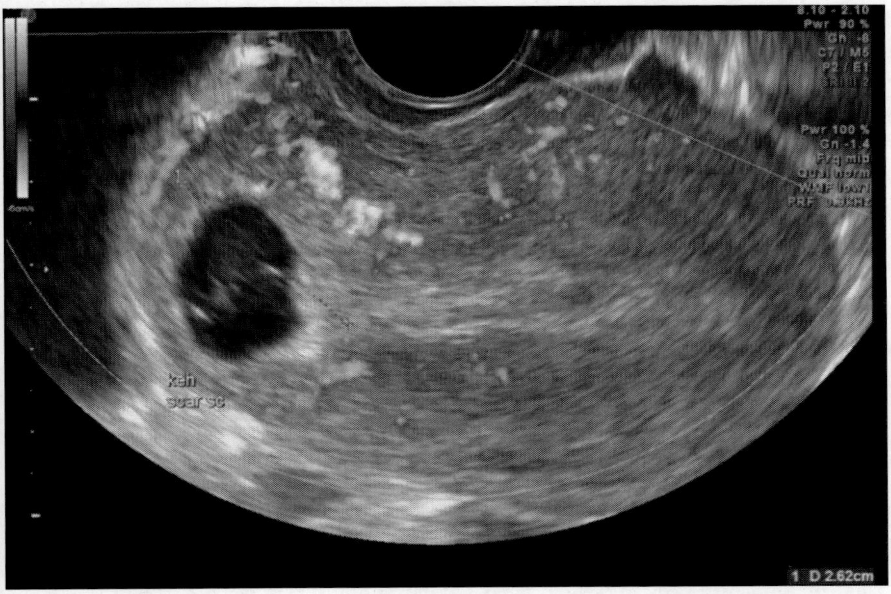

Figure 1. Ultrasound finding of cesarean scar pregnancy before administration of methotrexate. A gestational sac with a diameter of 2.62 cm was seen.

The patient had reported spotting in the previous 2 weeks, but the midwife said that the fetus was not developed; therefore, she visited the Department of Obstetrics and Gynecology where she was diagnosed with a CSP. She had no abdominal pain, nausea, or vomiting. Urination and defecation were within normal limits. Her beta-human chorionic gonadotropin (β-hCG) levels at the time of presentation were 34,968.12 mIU/mL. The patient was carefully counseled for both medical and surgical options; she refused to undergo surgery. After confirmation of a normal complete blood count (CBC) and normal liver/renal function test results, methotrexate 50 mg/m^2 was administered as a single dose via intravenous infusion according to the "two-dose regimen" of methotrexate published by Barnhart et al. in 2007 [7]. The second dose was given 4 days after the first dose; β-hCG levels decreased to 23,120.66 mIU/mL, and transvaginal ultrasound revealed that the gestational sac had become smaller (Figure 2).

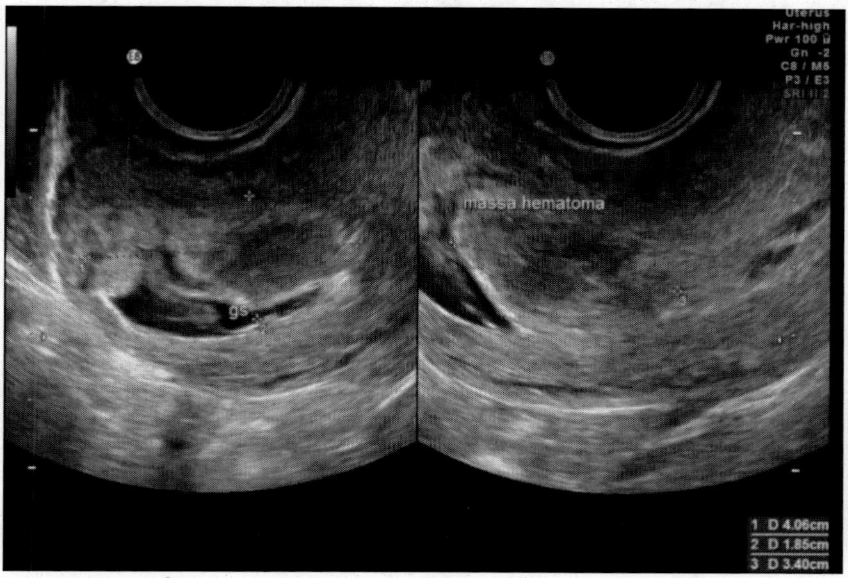

Figure 2. Ultrasound finding of cesarean scar pregnancy after administration of methotrexate.

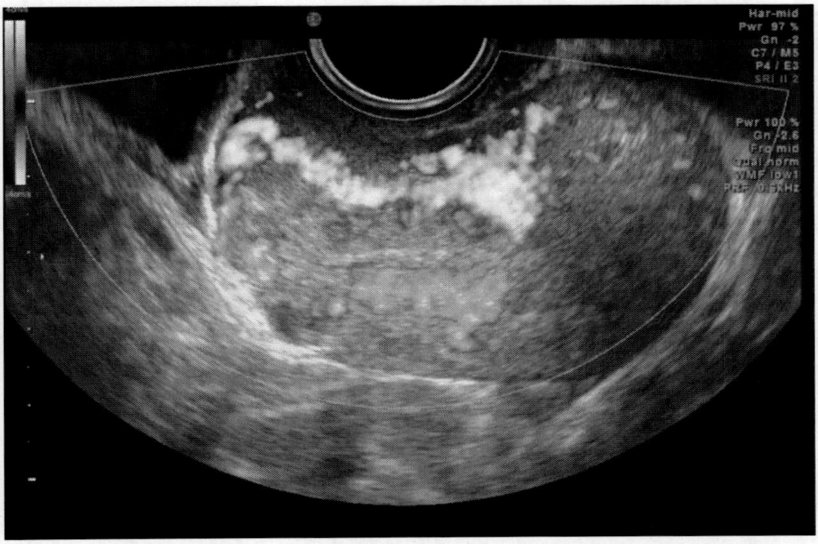

Figure 3. Ultrasound image showing the absence of the gestational sac, with 16 × 16 × 14 mm of the remaining conception tissue in the cesarean scar area.

Three days after the procedure, β-hCG levels had decreased to 14,164.00 mIU/mL, a decline of approximately 38%. Thereafter, the levels were measured weekly. During follow-up, the patient presented to the policlinic 1 week after with no complaint. The ultrasound revealed the absence of the gestational sac, with 16 × 16 × 14 mm of the remnant conception tissue (Figure 3); β-hCG levels on the same day had dropped to 996.88 mIU/mL.

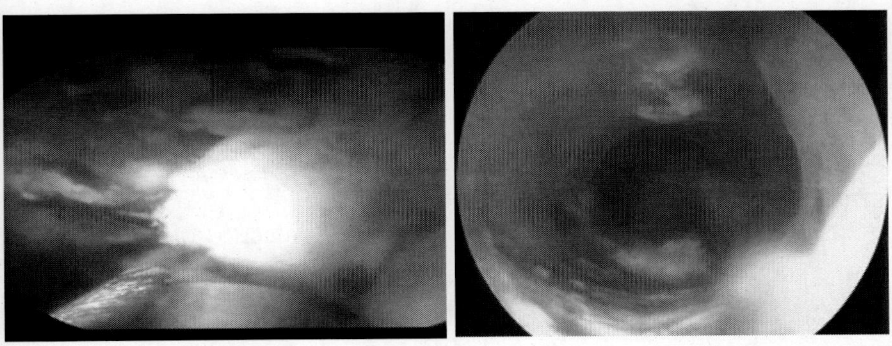

(a) (b)

Figure 4. Hysteroscopic Procedure (a) before the Procedure and (b) After the Procedure.

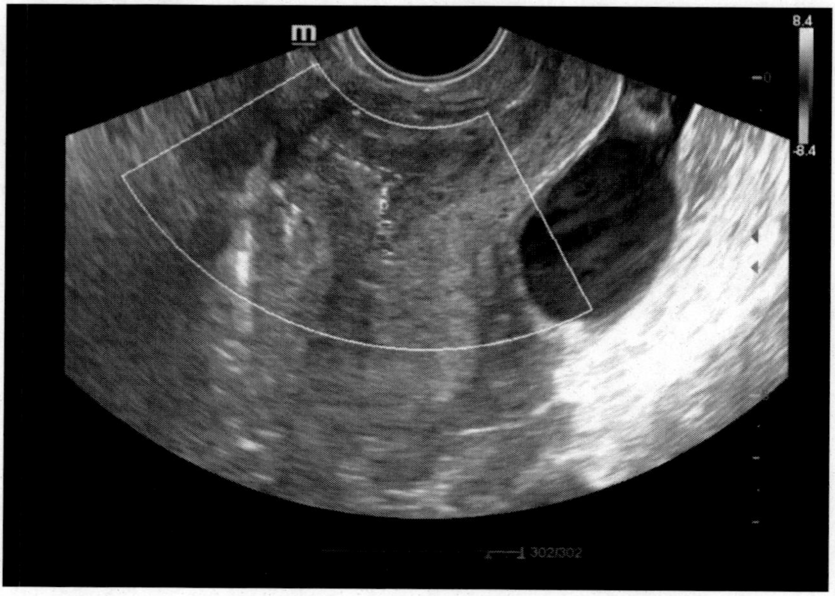

Figure 5. Ultrasound finding after the hysteroscopic procedure.

The CBC and blood chemistry results were within normal limits. We expected a decrease in β-hCG levels following two doses of methotrexate. Seven days later, β-hCG levels had decreased to 251.29 mIU/mL, and a hysteroscopic procedure was performed (Figure 4). Following the procedure, the remnant tissue was removed, and it was no longer seen on ultrasound (Figure 5).

DISCUSSION

There are many options for treating CSP. The options were surgical and medical treatment. The medical treatment such as injection of methotrexate and the surgical treatment are more invasive ranging from the resection of the uterine by using hysteroscopic modalities to more invasive procedure such as hysteroscopic resection of the mass [1]. This patient refused the surgery and preferred a less and minimal invasive procedure. We treated the patient by using methotrexate and combination with minimal invasive procedure.

The successful rate of using systemi methotrexate alone ranging from 57-100%, the recommendation was based on the selest cases of tubal ectopic pregnancy [5]. The possibility of the variation occurred due to the differences of the dense, fibrotic tissue that inhibit the penetration of methotrexate [5]. Another possible explanation is protocol combination of the CSP treatment. Lam et al. [8] review the factors that may lead the failure of treatment in using methotrexate alone. There is a 25% failure report but no common factor have been identified.

Since the cases of CSP are not many, the factors that lead to the failure of using methotrexate alone to treat CSP was not easy to be found. This treatment protocol was given to those patients who wish to not do surgery, and have no contraindication to methotrexate theraphy. Barnhart et al. stated that "*a third or fourth dose of methotrexate could be given in accordance with the "two-dose regimen" of methotrexate*" [7]. If the β-hCG levels decrease to 15% or more from the previous evaluation, weekly follow up of β-hCG level is needed until the level reach to less that 1 mIU/ml. Surgical intervention is conducted if the patient showed instability of hemodynamic or severe abdominal pain after the dose of methotrexate was given [9]. We would also consider surgical intervention if β-hCG levels continue to rise even after four doses of systemic methotrexate, fetal heart beat is still present, the are increase in size of the geatational mas. In our patient, β-hCG levels declined by 38% following the two-dose regimen, and therefore, the treatment was considered to be successful (Table 1).

Table 1. Beta-human chorionic gonadotropin (β-hCG) levels from day 0 to day 21 after the first methotrexate dose

No.	Date	β-hCG (mIU/mL) levels	Day	β-hCG reduction (%)
1	3/1/19	34,968	0	
2	7/1/19	23,120	4	33
3	10/1/19	14,164	7	38
4	17/1/19	996	14	92
5	23/1/19	251	21	74

This case is an important contribution to the research on CSP treatment. Our use of systemic methotrexate followed by a hysteroscopic procedure using an IBS is an example of a safe and effective conservative therapy for terminating a first-trimester CSP while preserving the woman's fertility.

REFERENCES

[1] Rotas, M., Haberman, S., Levgur, M., (2006). Cesarean Scar Ectopic Pregnancies: Etiology, Diagnosis, and Management. *Obstet. Gynecol,* 107: 1373-1381.

[2] Santos-Ribeiro, S., Tournaye, H., Polyzos, N. P., (2016). Trends in ectopic pregnancy rates following assisted reprodutive technologies in the UK: a 12-year nationwide analysis including 160000 pregnancies. *Hum. Reprod,* 31:393-402.

[3] World Health Organization and Human Reproduction Programme. (2015). *WHO statement on caesarean section rates: Executive summary*. Available from: https://www.who.int/reproductivehealth/ publications/ maternal_perinatal_health/cs-statement/en/.

[4] Rheinboldt, M., Osborn, D., Delproposto, Z., (2015). Cesarean section scar ectopic pregnancy: a clinical case series. *J. Ultrasound*, 18: 191-195.

[5] Riaz, R., Williams, T. R., Craig, B. M., Myers, D. T., (2015). Cesarean scar ectopic pregnancy: imaging, features, current treatment options, and clinical outcomes. *Abdom. Imaging*, 40: 2589-2599.

[6] Pirjani, R., Bayani, L., Shirazi, M., (2015). Successful local and systemic medical treatment of cesarean scar pregnancy and a subsequent term pregnancy after treatment: a case series. *Iran. J. Reprod. Med,* 13: 445-450.

[7] Barnhart, K., Hummel, A. C., Sammel, M. D., Menon, S., Jain, J., Chakhtoura, N., (2007). Use of "2-dose" regimen of methotrexate to treat ectopic pregnancy. *Fertil. Steril,* 87: 250-256.

[8] Lam, P., Lo, K., Lau, T., (2004). Unsuccessful medical treatment of cesarean scar ectopic pregnancy with systemic methotrexate: a report of two cases. *Acta. Obstet. Gynecol. Scand,* 83: 108-111.

[9] Schufreider, A., (2016). Successful termination of a cesarean scar ectopic pregnancy with systemic methotrexate and local potassium chloride injection. *J. Reprod. Endocr,* 1: 2-8.

[10] Veerbeek JH, Nikkels PG, Torrance HL, Gravesteijn J, Post Uiterweer ED, Derks JB, et al. (2014). Placental pathology in early intrauterine growth restriction associated with maternal hypertension. *Pubmed,* 35(9): 696–701.

[11] Salafia CM, Vogel CA, Vintzileos AM, Bantham KF, Pezzullo J, Silberman L. (1991). Placental pathologic findings in preterm birth. *Am J Obstet Gynecol,* 165(4 Pt 1):934–938. [PubMed: 1951558].

n: Obstetric and Gynecology Case Report ISBN: 978-1-53616-711-5
Editor: Dwiana Ocviyanti

Chapter 8

HOLISTIC MANAGEMENT IN OBSTETRIC CASES

Dwiana Ocviyanti[1], Lili Widjaya[2,*] and Kristian Alda[2]

[1]Department of Obstetric and Gynecology, Faculty of Medicine, Universitas Indonesia, Dr. Cipto Mangunkusumo Hospital, Jakarta, Indonesia

[2]Faculty of Medicine, Universitas Indonesia, Jakarta, Indonesia

ABSTRACT

Based on a population survey conducted in 2015, the maternal mortality rate in Indonesia was 305 per 100,000 live births. Hence, holistic management is needed to reduce maternal and infant mortality to achieve the target set as part of Sustainable Development Goals. Aside from comprehensive and accurate management, clinicians should propose a management strategy that involves an interprofessional approach to manage the patients optimally. This study aims to discuss holistic management in obstetric patients who require interprofessional management based on their biopsychosocial aspects. This case series

---

* Corresponding Author's E-mail: drliliwidjaya10@gmail.com.

reported 18 patients with an obstetric issue who were admitted to Dr. Cipto Mangunkusumo General Hospital in 2018-2019. The inclusion criterion is obstetric cases that emphasize biopsychosocial management. In 2018-2019, we encountered 7 cases of adolescent pregnancy, 2 cases of preeclampsia, 3 cases of preterm labor, 2 cases of abortion on unwanted pregnancy, 1 case of unwanted pregnancy with carcinoma on chemoradiation, 1 case of wanting pregnancy during an end-stage disease, 1 case of pregnancy on neglected people, and 1 case of unwanted pregnancy because of economic problem. Holistic and comprehensive management are needed for obstetric patients to reduce maternal and infant mortality. Holistic management included biopsychosocial aspect.

Keywords: holistic, obstetric case, maternal and infant, mortality

INTRODUCTION

Maternal and infant mortality are a serious and urgent problem in Indonesia. The results of Millennium Development Goals show that the reduction in maternal mortality is still very far from the target of 305/100,000–102/100,000 live births [1]. This situation needs to be paid attention to. The newborn mortality rate is also high, although it had reduced from 19/1000 in 2012 to 15/1000 live births in 2017 [1, 2].

Many factors contribute to the high maternal and infant mortality rates in Indonesia. Some of these factors are high anemia rate in pregnant females (48.9%), consistently low hospital birth rates (33%), high teenage pregnancy rate, low educational attainment of mothers in Indonesia, unsatisfactory economic levels, and other medical problems [3]. Based on *Data Rutin Direktorat Bina Kesehatan Ibu* in 2015, medical conditions that caused maternal deaths in Indonesia are as follows: bleeding (31%), hypertension (26%), and the rest (43%) comprising infections, metabolic disorders, bleeding disorders, and other diseases [4]. Therefore, this study aims to individually describe the selected obstetric cases in terms of their holistic and comprehensive management.

CASE REPORTS

Case 1

A 17-year-old female presented to the emergency department with fetal distress in the second stage of labor and early premature rupture of membranes (33 weeks' gestation). A difference was noted with respect to the gestational age mentioned by the patient between the first day of her last menstruation and the estimated fetal weight during the initial examination. However, after the fundal height, maximal cervical dilatation, and fetal distress were confirmed, vacuum extraction was performed. Then, the infant (weight 3000 g) was delivered successfully. As confirmed by the Ballard Score, the infant was 40 weeks old. The patient underwent IUD insertion postpartum. After the physician investigated the patient's history thoroughly, it was found that the patient conceived before marriage and had never undergone antenatal examination. The patient also stated that her parents are divorced, and her friends at school bullied her. Eventually, she and her boyfriend got unregistered married that was forced by their family.

Case 2

An unmarried 19-year-old female, who was pregnant for the first time, approached the emergency room with intrauterine fetal death and hypovolemic shock due to antepartum bleeding caused by placental abruption. She did not disclose her pregnancy to her parents because she was scared of being lambasted. Hence, she never underwent antenatal check-ups (ANCs). Furthermore, she had no health insurance and her boyfriend unemployed. Upon general examination, it was found that the patient had pale conjunctiva and cold extremities and was underweight [body mass index (BMI): 16.89 kg/m^2]. Obstetric examination revealed that her uterine fundal height (UFH) was 28 cm with tetanic contractions. In addition, the fetus weighed approximately 2325 g, with no fetal heart rate (FHR). Ultrasound results indicated that the placenta was attached to the uterine side wall. Laboratory examination revealed that the hemoglobin concentration was 5.8 gr/dl, and the platelet count was 36,000. Thus, the patient was diagnosed with hypovolemic shock owing to bleeding caused by placental abruption. Parents agreed to have the patient admitted for undergoing cesarean section and partial hysterectomy, considering that the situation could endanger patient's life. Treatments provided were as follows: uterotonic administration, blood transfusion, and HCU treatment. The patient was discharged on the third day. However, the family was concerned that the patient will not be able to conceive again.

Case 3

16-year-old female was referred to RSCM for fetomaternal ultrasound at 26 weeks' gestation at G1P0A0. This single live fetus was suspected of having omphalocele rupture. The patient often had sexual intercourse with her boyfriend, whom she met on Facebook. Both of them were high school students. Her parents had a divorce because of her father's physical abuse toward her mother. Since then, her mother got married thrice. The patient and her boyfriend finally quit school and got unregistered married. The husband worked in a car wash station. At 39 weeks gestation, the patient felt contractions; hence, cesarean section was performed. Unfortunately, the infant died 3 days later.

Case 4

A 17-year-old female was 36 weeks pregnant with a single live fetus with breech presentation accompanied by reduced amniotic fluid, preeclampsia, restricted fetal growth, and underweight. Considering these characteristics, the patient underwent cesarean section, and the infant was born at 1450 g in weight. According to the Ballard Score, the infant was 32–34 weeks old. During pregnancy, the patient had been treated with amniotic fluid transfusion and lung maturation. The patient was unmarried. Although her family supported her pregnancy, she remained depressed.

Case 5

An 18-year-old female, who was pregnant for the second time, approached the hospital at 35 weeks' gestation. The patient had a single live fetus with head presentation and had a history of SC once as well as candidiasis and iron deficiency anemia. She routinely had her pregnancy checked; thus, recurrence of anemia was known. At 33–34 weeks gestation, the fetal weight was low (1900 g); however, the fetus was healthy. Moreover, the patient had been married for 8 months; her husband worked as a taxi driver with a salary of 3.5 million rupiah per month.

Case 6

15-year-old female came to the hospital with premature rupture of membranes 10 hours prior to consultation. The patient only had ANC once; hence, she never underwent ultrasound examination. Physical and laboratory examinations revealed stable hemodynamics, no contractions, and hemoglobin level of 9.7 mg/dl. Ultrasound results, which were obtained at 34 weeks gestation, indicated no anatomic abnormalities, an estimated fetal weight of 1500 g, and oligohydramnios. Cesarean section was performed, and the infant was delivered successfully with a birth weight of 1700 g and an Apgar score of 7/8. According to the patient's history, she was expelled from middle school, so she joined the motorcycle gang and often had sexual intercourse with her boyfriend. Then, she unofficially married her boyfriend when she was 6 months pregnant. Her husband worked as "pengamen ondel-ondel" with an income around 35,000/day.

Case 7

An unmarried 17-year-old female came to the hospital at 4 months pregnant. The patient was still in high school. She confessed that she had sexual intercourse with her boyfriend twice without contraception, and she took a herbal medicine to resume her menstruation. After taking the medicine, ruptured membranes and spotting occurred. Though she had an episode of nausea, her vital signs and physical examination were normal. In the obstetric examination, the external ostium was dilated for approximately 2 cm. Ultrasound examination revealed a single fetus without FHR and with dry amniotic fluid. Patients diagnosed with intrauterine fetal death due to abortion at 18 weeks of her first pregnancy, indicative of juvenile and unwanted pregnancy. Then, misoprostol was administered to aid in fetal expulsion. She was also given antibiotic injection for her treatment and underwent psychiatric and forensic consultation.

Case 8

A 20-year-old female at 32 weeks pregnant (G1P0A0) complained of contractions and spotting. The patient only had ANC once and never had an ultrasound examination. The patient had been a commercial sex worker since 2 years ago. She confessed that she often had sexual intercourse with other males even during pregnancy. Her boyfriend ran away and stole her money. She did not have identification card and health insurance. She also never contacted or communicated with her family. During physical assessment, the FHR was 90 beats per minute (BPM) during contractions or not. Cesarean section was then performed. The infant was born, weighing 1850 g. After being treated for several days, the patient cannot be discharged because of inability to settle the hospital bills. Hence, the church paid for her bill and provided her a place to stay.

Case 9

A 20-year-old female came to the hospital with vaginal bleeding. The patient said that she was 5 months pregnant and not yet married. She did not want this pregnancy, so she attempted to abort the fetus by taking 6 tablets of misoprostol (3 tablets intravaginally and 3 tablets orally). She purchased the misoprostol on the Internet. After 4 hours of taking the medicine, the infant was born in her bathroom. Physical and laboratory examination results were within normal limits. In the obstetric examination, the umbilical cord was expulsed intravaginally, the placenta was felt on external uterine ostium, vaginal was not bleeding, and cervical was dilated 2 cm. Then stage III labor management was performed. Thereafter, this case was handled by the police.

Case 10

A 36-year-old female came to the hospital complaining of contraction. She said that she was 8 months pregnant, but she forgot the first day of her last menstruation. Since the beginning of her pregnancy, the patient, who was an active smoker, had been experiencing cough. In addition, she had a history of pulmonary tuberculosis (TB); nevertheless, the treatment was completed. Unfortunately, her husband died from TB. The patient worked as a parking attendant and a scavenger daily with irregular income. With an inadequate income, her children helped out as panhandlers. They lived in a 3 × 2-meter house, which was made of carton. In addition, she did not have an identification card. Physical examination revealed an increased respiration rate of 23 cycles per minute (CPM) with positive crackles in both lung fields. During the obstetric examination, a 26 cm of fundal height was obtained, with a fetal head presentation, Hodge 5/5, existing contractions, a FHR of 157 BPM, an estimated fetal weight of 1860 g, and a dilated external ostium. Furthermore, the laboratory examination showed that the leukocyte count was 10.100/µl. Appropriate management was provided, and it included contraction prevention, pulmonary maturation, antibiotic administration, and lung consultation with a plan to check the Acid-Fast

Bacillus Testing and chest X-ray. She was then planned for a long-term contraception. Furthermore, DKI Jakarta social service will take care of her.

Case 11

A 34-year-old female, who was 12 weeks pregnant (G5P3A1) came to the hospital for abortion due to unwanted and unplanned pregnancy. The patient did not want her pregnancy because of financial difficulty. Her second child needed an epilepsy treatment, which costs around 1.2 million Rupiah each month. Currently, the patient is still breastfeeding her third child. Furthermore, her husband had been unemployed since 2 years ago. Currently, patient works at the National Narcotics Agency, with a salary of 5 million Rupiah per month. After giving birth to her third child, she had asked for tubectomy. However, at that time, the labor was normal, and the patient returned without contraception. The patient had a history of toxoplasma with positive antitoxoplasma IgG and negative IgM. Other physical examinations were within normal limits.

Case 12

A 24-year-old female came to the hospital, with the desire to get pregnant. The patient had been married for 3 years and was still in a regular sexual contact. At present, she was diagnosed with stage 5 Chronic Kidney Disease and had undergone routine hemodialysis twice weekly since 2 years ago. The patient was pregnant before, but the infant died, with a premature weight of 900 g. At that time, the patient had preeclampsia. She had a history of taking antihypertensive medications, such as amlodipine, bisoprolol, and valsartan. Her father also had hypertension. Currently, the patient was not working, but her husband worked with 3.5 million Rupiah monthly income. Physical examination results showed a blood pressure of 170/100 mmHg, anemic conjunctiva, cardiomegaly, and positive systolic and diastolic murmurs. Moreover, the urea/creatinine level was 135/11.4, the echocardiogram indicated that she had a Congestive Heart Failure (CHF) with Ejection Fraction (EF) 34%, and the chest X-ray confirmed the occurrence of cardiomegaly. Hence, the patient was diagnosed with primary infertility for 3 years, anemia, hypertension, subclavian venous stenosis, and CHF FC II with EF 34%. Management was provided in accordance with the Internist and cardiovascular thoracic surgeons colleagues, and a conference will be held regarding the patient's preference for pregnancy.

Case 13

A 25-year-old female presented with a complaint of premature rupture of membrane for 2 weeks and was diagnosed with Preterm Premature Rupture of Membrane (PPROM) 14 days at 19 weeks gestation (G1P0A0). Her pregnancy consisted of a single fetus with severe oligohydramnios. Previously, the patient was control at clinic, and considering that no intrauterine infection was observed, the doctor advised her to take the prescribed medication and hydrate with 5 liters of fluids daily for 2 weeks. She and her family had been eagerly waiting for this pregnancy. However, after considering the advice from perinatology and the fetomaternal-related poor prognosis, the patient decided to terminate the pregnancy. The patient was unemployed, and her husband was a factory employee with an income of 4 million Rupiah per month.

Case 14

A 33-year-old female who was 33 weeks pregnant came to the hospital with 3-hour premature rupture of membrane. The Vital sign examination revealed the blood pressure was 180/110, the pulse rate was 100 BPM, and the respiratory rate was 24 CPM. Furthermore, general examination revealed no abnormalities. In the obstetric examination, 42 cm of fundal height, no contraction, and FHR were found. Amniotic fluid discharge was not noted, and the external ostium was not dilated. As depicted in the ultrasound, 1680,

1672, and 1669 g of fetal weight were found, and no perfusion abnormalities were found in the fetuses. Laboratory tests were within normal limits. However, the patient was diagnosed with impending eclampsia at 33 weeks pregnant with 3 live fetuses. The patient then received nifedipine, $MgSO_4$, and dexamethasone therapy and terminated the pregnancy with Cesarean Section (C-Section). Previously, the patient had given birth once, but the infant died of congenital heart disease.

Case 15

A 29-year-old female, who was 24 weeks pregnant, was diagnosed with left maxillary squamous cell carcinoma (T4bN0Mx) and received cisplatin chemotherapy. A joint conference agreed that the patient would continue her chemoradiation therapy, and C- Section would be administered after chemoradiation. C-Section was performed because the patient had Human Immunodeficiency Virus (HIV) without Antiretroviral (ARV). Preterm baby weighing 2100 g was born and treated at the Neonatal Intensive Care Unit (NICU) because of preterm complications. This pregnancy was undesirable. The patient's boyfriend was a mine worker with unknown HIV status. Her boyfriend also had a history of sexual intercourse with multiple partner.

Case 16

A 15-year-old teenager (G1P0A0) in the 11 weeks pregnant came to the hospital with vaginal bleeding. Her vital signs were within normal limits, BMI was 25.8 kg/m^2, the uterus was at the umbilical level, the portio was smooth, and the external ostium was closed with no flux. As shown on the ultrasound, a vesicular avascular mass measuring 139 × 54 mm was detected. Stratum basalis from endometrium was regular without invasion. Endocervix and portio were normal. No abnormal mass was found on either adnexa. The patient was then diagnosed with hydatidiform mole. Chest X-ray was normal, and results of the laboratory examination were as follows:

hemoglobin level 12.1 g/dl; B-hCG level 957.790 IU/L. Suction curettes were performed, and B-hCG level decreased to 90,393 IU/L.

According to the patient's history, she was forced by her parents to marry by increasing her age on her identification card because her parents were ashamed of her getting pregnant out of wedlock. Her 28-year-old husband worked as a driver with an income of 50,000 Rupiah per day. She was dropped out of high school. Furthermore, she never met her biological father. She is also a child who born from unmarital parents. Then she underwent psychiatric consultation to receive supportive psychotherapy because of adjustment problems.

Case 17

A 27-year-old nurse came to the hospital when she was 9 months pregnant (G1P0A0). During pregnancy, the patient underwent ANC regularly at the hospital and gained 16.9 kg. She had no history of hypertension before or during pregnancy. However, her blood pressure increased up to 126/80 mmHg during pregnancy with negative proteinuria. Her mother had a history of hypertension, during physical examination, her blood pressure was found to be 170/100 mmHg, but her general condition was within normal limit. In addition, the cervix was still immature. Her laboratory results revealed +1 urine protein. She was diagnosed as having preeclampsia with severe features. Then her pregnancy was terminated using 25 μg of vaginal misoprostol. When observation, she also complained of headache and nausea. Subsequently, she was diagnosed with impending eclampsia. The termination was continued with C-Section. A live baby girl was born with an Apgar score of 6/8, body weight of 2900 g, and body length of 46 cm. After treatment, the mother and the infant were discharged in good condition.

Case 18

A 34-year-old female came to the hospital with complaints of severe shortness of breath and Intra Uterine Fetal Death (IUFD) at term pregnancy. Her blood pressure was 220/110 mmHg; $MgSO_4$ was administered. The patient never underwent ANC because it requires payment, and she had no health insurance. She had completed junior high school, whereas her husband had completed elementary school. On physical examination, it was found that she experienced somnolence and gasping, oxygen saturation was 76%, BMI was 24.9 kg/m^2, blood pressure was 156/100 mmHg, and crackles were noted in both lung fields. Results of obstetric examination revealed complete cervical opening, fetal head presentation with Hodge III-IV, and baby weighing estimation of 3100 g; no FHR was detected on ultrasound or physical examination. Patient was diagnosed with second-stage labor at G1P0A0, aterm, fetal head presentation with IUFD, preeclampsia with severe features, and acute respiratory failure owing to pulmonary edema. The management provided was stabilization, intubation, acceleration of labor by using forceps extraction, and ICU care. After delivery, the patient was treated for 2 days in the ICU, and the blood pressure was 100/70 mmHg on the sixth day of treatment.

Discussion

Nowadays, it is globally accepted that health and illness are the outcome of an interaction between biopsychosocial factors. So that biological, psychological, and social aspect are needed in the healthcare management [5]. Biopsychosocial factors which are included in a holistic approach are very important in management of obstetric patients. In this case series we got 18 cases which can be classified into several problems such as adolescent pregnancy, abortion, unwanted pregnancy, pregnancy on neglected people, preterm labor, preeclampsia, and woman with end-stage disease with desire to get pregnant.

Pregnancy among 15-19 years old woman has a three-fold risk of death compared to 20-24 years old. Adolecents pregnancy are more susceptible to occur premature delivery, low birth weigh babies, fistula, and obstructed labor than women with older age [6].

Some of the adolescent pregnancy problems that occur in this case series were fetal distress, intrauterine fetal death, restricted fetal growth, placental abruption, premature rupture of membranes, preeclampsia, and hybdatidiform mole. Some of them got C-Section and even partial hysterectomy.

Most teenagers experienced unwanted pregnancies because they were not married. Consequently, they were forced to marry by her parents. Some of them got psychological problem such as depression and adjustment disorder. In this case series, one teenager who occured unwanted pregnancy decided to abort her pregnancy which lead to criminal action. Yussif et al. study revealed that at first pregnancy, teenagers < 19 years old have a higher risk (37%) to have an abortion compared to older women [7].

Mostly pregnancy in teenager are unwanted pregnancies. So that the teenagers did not pay attention to their health during pregnant. Some of them did not do ANC or only go few times. The absence of health insurance also caused that problem.

From the social aspect, teenagers who are pregnant will be bullied by their friends and their environment. Some teenagers dropped out of school because they were ashamed. In addition, the father of the child also had stopped from school because he had to work. The income earned were also low due to the educational background and inadequate skills. From these cases we learn that the management not only depends on patient illness but also other aspects such as psychological, social, and financial problem.

Beside of these adolescent pregnancies, we also got unwanted pregnancy cases which were caused by financial problem and unmarried pregnancy. One of these case leads to abortion by using drugs which were purchased on the internet.

We also got one case about pregnancy in woman with neglected status. She lives in an inappropriate place that it could affect her health. During pregnancy she had been cought that were suspected pulmonary TB.

Beside of biological aspect, psychological and social aspect also need to consider as important thing. Her husband died because of pulmonary TB. She also had history of this disease. Somehow, she must worry about her condition and her children health.

For living, she worked as parking attendant and a scavenger with irregular income. Her children helped out as panhandlers. She is a single parent who have to take care of her children. In this cases, social service was very needed to help her and her family.

We got several cases about preeclampsia. One of them occured in 34 years old woman who was diagnosed with second-stage labor at G1P0A0, aterm, fetal head presentation with IUFD, preeclampsia with severe features, and acute respiratory failure owing to pulmonary edema. The patient never went to ANC so that preeclampsia was not detected. Factors such as first pregnancy, obesity, and the absence of antenatal visits should be identified as risk factors for preeclampsia. This is in line with English et al. study that revealed nullipara, obesity, family history, diabetes and egg donation as a multiple risk factors for preeclampsia. Prevention, early detection and treatment are the effective management for preeclampsia [8]. Psychology aspect in this patient must be considered. Intrauterine fetal death was traumatic for the patient. Haezell et al. study revealed that stillbirth is associated with economic cost, psychological and social problem for parents. These conditions may affect the next pregnancies which already increased risk of the complication [9]. Many women who are experience with preeclampsia will have feeling close to death and fear [10]. That statement is very likely to happen considering the severe clinical condition of patient that was happened. Spritual care are needed for pregnant women with preeclampsia to reduce their risk of PTSD (Postpartum stress disorder) [11].

Social aspect on this patient must also be considered. The patient did not have health insurance, so she did not check her pregnancy. In the future the patient should be advised to have health insurance so that the financial problem would not cause severe complications on the patient health.

CONCLUSION

Holistic and comprehensive management are needed for obstetric patients to reduce maternal and infant mortality. Holistic management included biopsychosocial aspect.

REFERENCES

[1] Taher, A., et al. (2018). Evidence summit untuk mengurangi kematian ibu dan bayi baru lahir di indonesia: ringkasan eksekutif [Evidence summit to reduce maternal and newborn mortality]. *AIPI*: 18 p. Available from: https://aipi.or.id/frontend/report/read/424773415a773d3d

[2] Gustina, E. (2019). *Pengantar fokus grup diskusi strategi penurunan AKI dan AKN* [*Introduction of focus group discussion maternal and neonatal mortality rate*]. Ministry of Health Republic of Indonesia.

[3] Badan penelitian dan pengembangan kesehatan (Agency for health research and development). (2018). *Hasil utama riskesdas* [*The main outcome of basic health research*]. Ministry of Health Republic of Indonesia: 88 p. Available from: http://www.depkes.go.id/resources/download/info-terkini/materi_rakorpop_2018/Hasil%20Riskesdas%202018.pdf

[4] Ocviyanti, D. (2019). *Kematian Ibu di Indonesia dan Upaya Menurunkannya* [*Maternal mortality in Indonesia and the effort to reduce*]. Focus group discussion reducing maternal and neonatal mortality. Ministry of Health Republic of Indonesia.

[5] Wade, D. T. & Halligan, P. W. (2017). The biopsychosocial model of illness: a model whose time has come. *Clinical Rehabilitation*, 31(8): 995-1004. Available from: https://doi.org/10. 1177/0269215517709890

[6] Sedgh, G., et al. (2015). Adolescent pregnancy, birth, and abortion rates across countries: levels and recent trends. *Journal of adolescent*

health, *56* (2): 223-230. Available from: https://reader.elsevier.com/reader/sd/pii/ S1054139X14003875?token=02C01BE5CB58 B415E72D3096C5CB6D0FD37FBF7617A4AF544D4D6358BC1B625C68BF5E4B89427513766F41C25C827F7A

[7] Yussif, A. S., et al. (2017). The long term effects of adolescent pregnancies in a community in northern Ghana on subsequent pregnancies and births of young mothers. *Reproductive health*, *14* (178): 7p. Available from: https://reproductive-health-journal.biomedcentral.com/track/pdf/10.1186/ s12978-017-0443-x

[8] English, F. A., Kenny, L. C. & McCarthy, F. P. (2015). Risk factor and effective management of preeclampsia. *Dovepress journal*: 12 p. Available from: https://www.ncbi.nlm.nih.gov/pmc/articles/PMC4354613/ pdf/ibpc-8-007.pdf

[9] Heazell, A. P., et al. Care in pregnancies after stillbirth and perinatal death. *International journal of birth and parent education.* Available from: https://ijbpe.com/index.php/news/466-care-in-pregnancies-after-stillbirth-and-perinatal-death

[10] Vaerland, I. E., Vevatne, K. and Brinchmann, B. S. (2016). An integrative review of mother's experiences of preeclampasia. *Journal of obstetric*, *gynecologic & neonatal nirsing*, *45* (3): 300-307. Available from: https://www.sciencedirect.com/science/article/abs/pii/ S0884217516001647

[11] Kamali, Z., et al. (2018). Effect of spiritual care education on postpartum stress disorder in women with preeclampsia. *Journal of Education and Health Promotion. 7* (73): 43p. Available from: https://www.ncbi.nlm.nih. gov/pmc/articles/PMC6009134/

In: Obstetric and Gynecology Case Report
Editor: Dwiana Ocviyanti
ISBN: 978-1-53616-711-5

Chapter 9

AUTOIMMUNE HEPATITIS DURING PREGNANCY: OPTIMAL MANAGEMENT FOR DELIVERING AT TERM

Ali Sungkar, Raymond Surya*, Budi Iman Santoso, Surahman Hakim and Eka Rusdianto Gunardi
Department of Obstetrics and Gynecology, Faculty of Medicine, Universitas Indonesia, Dr. Cipto Mangunkusumo Hospital, Jakarta, Indonesia

ABSTRACT

Autoimmune hepatitis (AIH) is a chronic inflammatory disease characterized by progressive hepatocellular inflammation not related to alcohol consumption, viral infection, exposure to hepatotoxic drugs, or genetic liver disorders. AIH is associated with a high rate of miscarriage, stillbirth, and premature delivery. This study aimed to discuss the optimal management of AIH during pregnancy in order to maintain the pregnancy up to term. We also determined whether pregnancy influences the flare-up

* Corresponding Author's Email: raymond_s130291@yahoo.co.id.

of AIH or vice versa and what the best treatment for AIH during pregnancy is. The case illustration is a 32-year-old pregnant woman diagnosed with AIH delivered a healthy baby vaginally at 38 weeks of gestational age. The treatment strategy for AIH is to obtain complete remission and avoid further progression of the disease. The European Association for the Study of the Liver (EASL) states that the first-line therapy for AIH is prednisone/prednisolone, followed by the addition of azathioprine after 2 weeks. It can be concluded that optimal management of AIH during pregnancy is required in order to maintain the pregnancy up to term.

Keywords: autoimmune hepatitis, pregnancy, management, prednisolone, azathioprine

INTRODUCTION

Autoimmune hepatitis (AIH) is a chronic inflammatory disease characterized by progressive hepatocellular inflammation not related to alcohol consumption, viral infection, exposure to hepatotoxic drugs, or genetic liver disorders [1]. Because of its rare and heterogeneous nature, AIH still is a major diagnostic and therapeutic challenge. The prevalence of AIG is between 16 and 18 cases per 100,000 population in Europe [2–4]. The prevalence varies by ethnicity, with Alaskan natives showing a high frequency of the disease and the North American aborigines showing greater severity [5]. These differences reflect genetic predisposition, indigenous etiological agents, pharmacogenomic mechanism, and socioeconomic reasons, such as delayed diagnosis [6].

AIH usually affects young women of childbearing age. Patients usually complain of oligomenorrhea, but better clinical management has led to an increase in the number of pregnancies. AIH is associated with a high rate of miscarriage, stillbirth, and premature delivery [7, 8]. The presence of esophageal varices increases the risk of bleeding during pregnancy, especially in the second half of gestation [9]. However, fetal outcomes are good, similar to cases of other autoimmune disorders [10]. This study aimed to discuss the optimal management of AIH during pregnancy in order to maintain the pregnancy up to term. We also answered the following questions: Can pregnancy influence the flare-up of AIH or vice versa? What is the best treatment for AIH during pregnancy?

CASE ILLUSTRATION

A 32-year-old pregnant woman was diagnosed with AIH. Around 2 months before pregnancy, she complained of icterus in her whole body, nausea, and hepatomegaly. Further investigation had nonreactive results for anti–hepatitis A virus (anti-HAV), hepatitis B virus surface antigen (HBsAg), and anti–hepatitis C virus (anti-HCV). Her aspartate transaminase/alanine transaminase (AST/ALT) ratio and alkaline phosphatase level were 4–5 and 6–8 times above the normal range, respectively, while her gamma-globulin transferase level was 40 times above the normal limit. Autoimmune antibodies such as antinuclear antibody (ANA) were positive, and anti–double stranded DNA (anti-dsDNA) was within the normal limit. Total bilirubin was often above the normal limit, while direct bilirubin seemed higher compared to indirect bilirubin. Ultrasound (US) examination showed an enlarged liver with a normal echogenic parenchyma, no vascular and bile duct dilatation, and no mass or cyst.

The patient's International Autoimmune Hepatitis Group (IAIHG) score was 6, including positive ANA (≥1:80), gamma-globulin level >1.1x the upper limit, and the absence of viral hepatitis. Therefore, she patient was diagnosed with AIH and was administered methylprednisolone, HP pro, and curcuma. A contrast abdominal computed tomography scan was planned; however, she got pregnant before this procedure could be performed. US examination of the fetus did not show any major abnormalities. Finally, the patient delivered a healthy baby boy vaginally at 38 weeks of gestational age; the baby weighed 2800 g.

DISCUSSION

The International Autoimmune Hepatitis Group (IAIHG) states that a score of ≥7 indicates definite AIH, while a score of ≥6 indicates probable AIH.[11] Histological examination is essential for making a diagnosis of AIH. Although the patient had a score of 6, we did not perform a histological examination because of her pregnancy, and she was diagnosed with definite AIH and treated accordingly.

Pregnancy is a homeostatic state in which the fetal tissue is not rejected by the mother. This phenomenon is caused by the high concentration of estrogen, which inhibits the immune response [12]. In addition, progesterone promotes T-helper 2 (Th2) cells and shows anti-inflammatory activity [13]. Studies have demonstrated modifications of the maternal autoimmune system, especially in T-cell and natural killer cell function. AIH is similar to rheumatoid arthritis, which is considered to be a T-cell-mediated and Th1-immune-response-driven disorder. During pregnancy, there is a shift from the Th1 to the Th2 response, so it is uncommon for AIH to flare-up during pregnancy. In AIH, type 1 cytokines predominate in the liver during active inflammation, while type 2 cytokines predominate in the liver during remission [14]. Westbrook et al. [10] showed that a flare-up in AIH activity occurs in 33% of pregnant patients, of which a majority (78%) show a flare-up in the postpartum period. This finding was consistent with another study, although the underlying mechanism is still unclear, and in accordance with the development of immunological tolerance in order to allow the mother to tolerate paternally derived antigens expressed by the fetus through regulatory T-cells [15]. In addition, the AIH flare-up during pregnancy is related to poor disease control and the absence of therapy during pregnancy, leading to increased risk of hepatic decompensation and increased need for neonatal admission to a special care unit [10].

One of the adverse pregnancy outcomes of AIH during pregnancy is premature delivery (11.8% of patients in Brazil) [16], but the cause is unknown. Schramm et al. [17] found that the presence of antibodies to soluble liver antigen/liver-pancreas antigen and Ro/SSA is statistically significant for adverse pregnancy outcomes. They found serious maternal complications in 9% of patients, including acute fulminant hepatitis in 1 patient and septic abortion in another patient, who eventually suffered from multiorgan failure and died. Terrabuio et al. [7] reported that 68.4% of pregnant AIH patients end up with liver cirrhosis and 7.8% have serious complications such as renal failure after an emergency cesarean section, vaginal bleeding and infection in the postpartum period, and variceal bleeding during the second trimester; however, no maternal mortalities were recorded.

The treatment strategy for AIH is to obtain complete remission and avoid further progression of the disease. The European Association for the Study of the Liver (EASL) states that the first-line therapy for AIH is prednisone/prednisolone, followed by the addition of immunosuppression therapy with azathioprine after 2 weeks [18]. According to the US Food and Drug Administration, prednisone is a category C drug that does not cross the placenta to a significant degree. It is not associated with teratogenic effects in humans and therefore is a drug of choice for AIH during pregnancy [19]. According to the EASL, azathioprine can be initiated regardless of whether bilirubin levels are <6 mg/dL (100 μmol/L). The initial dosage of azathioprine is 50 mg/dL, which is increased on the basis of toxicity and response, while the maintenance dose is 1–2 mg/kg [18]. However, the safety of azathioprine in pregnancy is debatable. In animal models, azathioprine causes skeletal abnormalities, cleft palate, hydrops fetalis, and hemopoetic abnormalities in the fetus. Babies of women taking azathioprine have lymphopenia, hypogammaglobulinemia, or thymic hypoplasia. Despite these adverse outcomes, azathioprine should be continued during pregnancy in order to maintain AIH remission in the mother. Immunosuppression therapy reduces flare-ups compared to AIH patients not on immunosuppression therapy. In addition, preterm labor is more common in AIH patients not on immunosuppression therapy [10].

Therefore, during pregnancy, AIH patients should be administered immunosuppression therapy for complete remission. In addition, good antenatal care should be taken to maintain pregnancy up to term.

Conclusion

AIH rarely flares up during pregnancy because of alteration of the immune response by estrogen and progesterone. Optimal management of AIH during pregnancy should be performed to maintain the pregnancy up to term.

References

[1] Krawitt, E. L. (2006). Autoimmune Hepatitis. *New England Journal of Medicine,* 354: 54-66.

[2] van Gerven, N. M. F., Verwer, B. J., Witte, B. I., van Erpecum, K. J., van Buuren, H. R., Maijers, I., Visscher, A. P., Verschuren, E. C., van Hoek, B., Coenraad, M. J. and Beuers, U. H. (2014). Epidemiology and clinical characteristics of autoimmune hepatitis in the Netherlands. *Scandinavian Journal of Gastroenterology,* 49: 1245-1254.

[3] Werner, M., Prytz, H., Ohlsson, B., Almer, S., Björnsson, E., Bergquist, A., Wallerstedt, S., Sandberg-Gertzén, H., Hultcrantz, R., Sangfelt, P. and Weiland, O. (2008). Epidemiology and the initial presentation of autoimmune hepatitis in Sweden, a nationwide study. *Scandinavian Journal of Gastroenterology*, 43: 1232-12340.

[4] Ngu, J. H., Bechly, K., Chapman, B. A., Burt, M. J., Barclay, M. L., Gearry, R. B. and Stedman, C. A. (2010). Population-based epidemiology study of autoimmune hepatitis, a disease of older women. *Journal of Gastroenterology and Hepatology,* 25: 1681-1686.

[5] Minuk, G., Liu, S., Kaita, K., Wong, S., Renner, E., Rempel, J. and Uhanova, J. (2008). Autoimmune hepatitis in a North American Aboriginal/First Nations population. *Canadian Journal of Gastroenterology and Hepatology,* 10: 829-834.

[6] Czaja, A. J. (2013). Autoimmune hepatitis in diverse ethnic populations and geographical regions. *Expert Review of Gastroenterology & Hepatology,* 7: 365-385.

[7] Terrabuio, D. R. B., Abrantes-Lemos, C. P., Carrilho, F. J. and Cançado, E. L. R. (2009). Follow-up of pregnant women with autoimmune hepatitis, the disease behavior along with maternal and fetal outcomes. *Journal of Clinical Gastroenterology*, 43: 350-356.

[8] Muratori, P., Loffreda, S., Muratori, L., Ferrari, R., Afandi, K., Cassani, F., Pappas, G., Lenzi, M. and Bianchi, F. B. (2002) Spontaneous remission of autoimmune hepatitis during pregnancy. *Digestive and Liver Disease*, 34: 608-609.

[9] López-Méndez, E. and Avila-Escobedo, L. (2006). Pregnancy and portal hypertension a pathology view of physiologic changes. *Annals of Hepatology,* 5: 219-223.

[10] Westbrook, R. H., Yeoman, A. D., Kriese, S. and Heneghan, M. A. (2012). Outcomes of pregnancy in women with autoimmune hepatitis. *Journal of Autoimmunity,* 38: J239-J244.

[11] Hennes, E. M., Zeniya, M., Czaja, A. J., Parés, A., Dalekos, G. N., Krawitt, E. L., Bittencourt, P. L., Porta, G., Boberg, K. M., Hofer, H., Bianchi, F. B., Shibata, M., Schramm, C., Eisenmann de Torres, B., Galle, P. R., McFarlane, I., Dienes, H. P., Lohse, A. W. and International Autoimmune Hepatitis Group. (2008). Simplified criteria for the diagnosis of autoimmune hepatitis. *Hepatology,* 48: 169-176.

[12] Yip, L., McCluskey, J. and Sinclair, R. (2006). Immunological aspects of pregnancy. *Clinics in Dermatology:*84-87.

[13] Buchel, E., Van Steenbergen, W., Nevens, F. and Fevery, J. (2002). Improvement of autoimmune hepatitis during pregnancy followed by flare-up after delivery. *The American Journal of Gastroenterology,* 97: 3160-3165.

[14] Clowse, M. E. B. (2007). Lupus activity in pregnancy. *Rheumatic Disease Clinics of North America,* 33: 237-252.

[15] Aluvihare, V. R., Kallikourdis, M., Betz and A. G. (2005). Tolerance, suppression and the fetal allograft. *Rheumatic Disease Clinics of North America,* 83: 88-96.

[16] Aragão, V. M. de F., Silva, A. A. M. da., Aragão, L. F de., Barbieri, M. A., Bettiol, H., Coimbra, L. C. and Ribeiro, V. S. (2004). Risk

factors for preterm births in São Luís, Maranhão, Brazil. *Cadernos de Saúde Pública,* 20: 57-63.

[17] Schramm, C., Herkel, J., Beuers, U., Kanzler, S., Galle, P. R. and Lohse, A. W. (2006). Pregnancy in autoimmune hepatitis, outcome and risk factors. *The American Journal of Gastroenterology,* 101: 556-560.

[18] European Association for the study of the liver. (2009). EASL clinical practice guidelines: management of cholestatic liver diseases. *Journal of Hepatology,* 51: 237-267.

[19] Braga, A. C., Vasconcelos, C. and Braga, J. (2016). Pregnancy with autoimmune hepatitis. *Gastroenterology and Hepatology from Bed to Bench,* 9: 220-224.

SECTION 2: REPRODUCTIVE AND INFERTILITY

In: Obstetric and Gynecology Case Report ISBN: 978-1-53616-711-5
Editor: Dwiana Ocviyanti

Chapter 10

ALERT IN CONTRACEPTIVE IMPLANT FAILURE: A CASE REPORT

Raymond Surya[1,*] and Yanto Kusnawara[2]

[1]Department of Obstetrics and Gynecology, Faculty of Medicine, Universitas Indonesia, Dr. Cipto Mangunkusumo Hospital, Jakarta, Indonesia.

[2]Department of Obstetrics and Gynecology, Faculty of Medicine, Universitas Indonesia, Koja Hospital, Jakarta, Indonesia

ABSTRACT

The progestin-only subdermal implant levonorgestrel is a very effective contraceptive with a failure rate of only 0.05% within the first year of typical use. We herein present the case of a patient with two-rod levonorgestrel failure after discontinuing anti-tuberculosis medication at a district hospital. A 24-year-old female, para 1, was referred to the obstetrics polyclinic due to a positive pregnancy test. She had a two-rod levonorgestrel implant (Indoplant©) for the last two years. Seven months before referral, she was treated with rifampicin for 5 months due to

* Corresponding Author's Email: raymond_s130291@yahoo.co.id.

suspicious tuberculous lymphadenitis. An intrauterine pregnancy of 8+1 weeks with a crown-rump length of 1.72 mm was identified, and the implant was removed. Levonorgestrel binds to albumin and sex hormone-binding globulin, and levonorgestrel correlates with body weight. Rifampicin is known to induce liver CYP3A4 and decrease the area under the concentration-time curve by 55%. Concomitant use of rifampicin can reduce contraceptive agent concentrations, increasing pregnancy risk. The recommendation in these patients is pregnancy continuation because the implant does not affect the progression of pregnancy.

Keywords: levonorgestrel, implant, pregnancy, anti-tuberculosis drug

INTRODUCTION

Two-rod levonorgestrel implant (Indoplant©) used in Indonesia was adopted from Jadelle©, which has been in use in the USA since 1996. The implant comprises two flexible cylindrical dimethylsiloxane copolymer cores enclosed in thin-walled silicone tubing [1]; each core contains 75 mg levonorgestrel. Mean daily *in vivo* release of levonorgestrel is 100 μg/day during the first month, followed by a decline to 40 μg/day at 12 months and approximately 30 μg/day at 24 months and beyond. Indoplant© was initially licensed for 3-year use, which was later extended to five years based on clinical studies.

This progestin-only subdermal implant is very effective, with failure rate of only 0.05% within the first year of typical use [2, 3]. In the original study of one-rod levonorgestrel implant (marketed as Implanon©), there were no failures resulting in pregnancies. However, studies in Australia [4] and France [5] reported pregnancy in situ as a consequence of implant failure. The contraceptive failure is associated with poor insertion technique, insertion at the wrong time during the menstrual cycle, drug interaction, product/method failure, and unknown factors [4]. The mechanisms of action of this implant are changes in cervical mucus, ovulation inhibition, and promotion of ovulatory dysfunction. Cervical mucus becomes viscous and scanty, whereas the inhibition of ovulation occurs in over 85% of the cycles in the first year of use. The ovulatory dysfunction is described as inadequate gonadotropin surge, which plays a major role in the maturation of oocyte; thus, the oocyte may not be capable of fertilization after follicular rupture [6, 7].

In this case report, we present the case of a patient who experienced two-rod levonorgestrel failure after discontinuation of anti-tuberculosis medication at a district hospital.

CASE REPORT

A 24-year-old female, para-1, was referred to the obstetrics polyclinic due to a positive pregnancy test. She was not expecting pregnancy as she had a two-rod levonorgestrel implant (Indoplant©); she stated that she did not get regular menstruation for the last two years but that she experienced nausea and vomiting two weeks before visiting the polyclinic. In her medical history, she developed a mobile, tender, and painless mass in the right sternocleidomastoid region approximately seven months ago and was diagnosed with tuberculous lymphadenitis by an ear/nose/throat specialist; she was initiated on rifampicin. Five months after the start of treatment, there was no change in size of the mass, and the histopathological examination of the excision biopsy performed by a general surgeon revealed chronic granulomatous inflammation, which could be due to *M. tuberculosis*.

On physical examination, the vital signs were stable, and the body mass index was normal (20.4 kg/m^2). There was a scar in the right sternocleidomastoid region, and the two-rod implant in the left upper arm was palpable. On ultrasound examination, an intrauterine pregnancy with a crown-rump length (CRL) of 1.72 mm was found, indicating an appropriate gestation age of 8^{+1} weeks. Therefore, the implant was removed at the same time knowing there was intrauterine pregnancy (Figures 1 & 2).

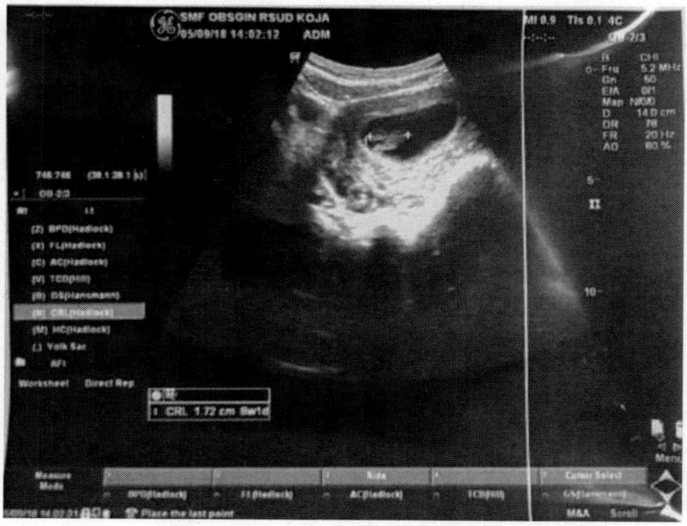

Figure 1. First-trimester intrauterine pregnancy.

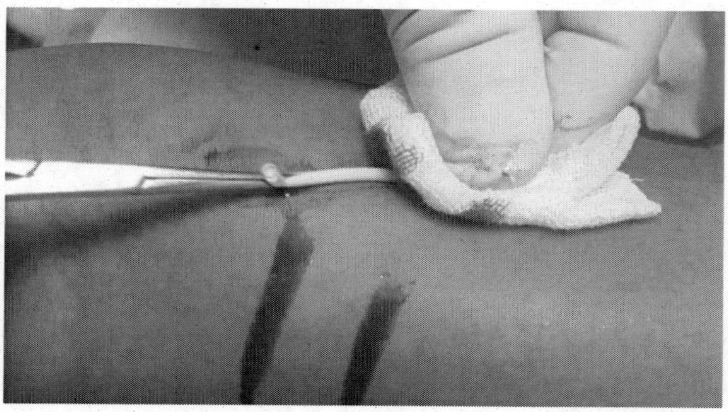

Figure 2. Implant removal.

Discussion

Levonorgestrel is delivered directly into the interstitial fluid from the subdermal implant. In serum, the drug is bound to albumin and sex hormone-binding globulin (SHBG), and approximately 1% to 2% of total serum levonorgestrel concentration is in free steroid. The secretion of SHBG, a glycoprotein, is induced by estrogen and suppressed by androgen; thus, levonorgestrel reduces SHBG concentration. Decreasing serum SHBG concentration will increase the fraction of unbound levonogestrel [8]. Maximum levonorgestrel concentration is reached in approximately 2–3 days, with mean and standard deviation of 772 and 414 pg/mL, respectively, on day 2. This is followed by a slow decline to 280 and 123 pg/mL at three years [1]. Irving et al. [9] found that the minimum levonorgestrel concentration for pregnancy prevention was below 200 pg/ml, even below 175 pg/ml. Additionally, levonorgestrel concentration correlates with body weight: total exposure of levonorgestrel decreases with increasing body weight between 39 and 160 kg [10]. The World Health Organization reported that pregnancy among women using the implant was rare for those weighing less than 70 kg at the time of implant insertion [11]. The current patient's body weight was less than 70 kg with an ideal body mass index (20.4 kg/m^2) so that this risk was minimalized.

The metabolism of levonorgestrel is affected by the enzyme cytochrome (CYP) P450 3A4, which is believed to be inactivated by ethinyl estradiol: the elimination rate of levonorgestrel was reduced in patients on combination oral contraception [10]. The elimination half-life is approximately 13 to 18 hours, and levonorgestrel is excreted mainly in the urine (40%–68%), whereas approximately 16%–48% is excreted in feces. After removal of the implant, levonorgestrel concentrations decrease below 100 pg/mL by 96 hours and below sensitivity between 5 days and 2 weeks [12].

One of the factors contributing to implant failure is drug interactions. Several medications with potent enzyme inducing effects have deleterious effects on hormonal contraceptives; these include antiepileptics (carbamazepine, phenytoin, phenobarbital, primidone, and topiramate), antibiotics (rifampicin, rifabutin), antifungals (griseofulvin), protease inhibitors (nelfinavir, ritonavir), and non-nucleoside reverse transcriptase inhibitors (efavirenz and nevirapine) [13]. In the current case, the cause of pregnancy was suspected to be the concomitant use of rifampicin as the anti-tuberculosis drug. Rifampicin is known to induce CYP3A4 in the liver, which is considered to reduce the plasma concentration of levonorgestrel.

Rifampicin can decrease 55% in the area under the concentration-time curve in pharmacokinetic drug interaction studies [14]. This effect explains the failure of contraception, which resulted in pregnancy. The medical eligibility criteria by the World Health Organization state that in patients treated with rifampicin, the first-line recommended contraception is depot medroxy-progesterone acetate (DMPA) (category I), followed by levonorgestrel or norethindrone enanthate (category II) and progestogen-only pill (category III) [15].

In the current case, the patient became pregnant due to contraceptive failure and did not desire abortion; therefore, she continued the pregnancy, and the implant was removed. It should be noted that there is no evidence of harm to the patient or the progression of pregnancy if the implant is not removed [16].

Conclusion

Concomitant use of rifampicin can reduce the concentration of contraceptive agents in implants, leading to pregnancy. In these patients, the recommendation is to continue pregnancy without removing the implant, which does not affect the progression of pregnancy.

References

[1] Rxlist. (2008). *JADELLE (levonorgestrel implants) for subdermal use*, 35. Available from: https://www.rxlist.com/jadelle-drug.htm#description.

[2] Moutchia-Suh, J., Mouemba, D. K. M. and Ngwasiri, C. A. (2018). Occurrence of anembryonic pregnancy with use of levonorgestrel subdermal implant (JADELLE®): a case report. *Journal of Medical Case Reports,* 12 (1): 111.

[3] Duvall, S., Thurston, S., Weinberger, M., Nuccio, O. and Fuchs-Montgomery, N. (2014). Scaling up delivery of contraceptive implants in sub-Saharan Africa: operational experiences of Marie Stopes International. *Global Health: Science and Practice,* 2 (1): 72-92.

[4] Harrison-Woolrych, M. and Hill, R. (2005). Unintended pregnancies with the etonogestrel implant (Implanon): a case series from postmarketing experience in Australia. *Contraception,* 71 (4): 306-308.

[5] Bensouda-Grimaldi, L., Jonville-Béra, A. P., Beau-Salinas, F., Llabres, S., Autret-Leca, E. and le réseau des centres régionaux de pharmacovigilance. (2005). Insertion problems, removal problems, and contraception failures with Implanon. *Gynécologie, obstétrique & fertilité,* 33 (12): 986-990.

[6] Brache, V., Alvarez, F. and Faundes, A. (2001). Mechanism of action of levonorgestrel contraceptive implants. *Gynecological Endocrinology,* 15 (II): 14-20.

[7] Mozzanega, B. and Cosmi, E. (2011). How do levonorgestrel-only emergency contraceptive pills prevent pregnancy? Some considerations. *Gynecological Endocrinology,* 27 (6): 439-442.

[8] Kuhnz, W., Schütt, B. and Woloszczak, R. (1994). Influence of changes in the concentration of sex hormone-binding globulin in human serum on the protein binding of the contraceptive steroids levonorgestrel, 3-keto-desogestrel and gestodene. *The Journal of Steroid Biochemistry and Molecular Biology,* 48 (5-6): 573-80.

[9] Sivin, I., Lähteenmäki, P., Ranta, S., Darney, P., Klaisle, C., Wan, L., Mishell, D. R. Jr., Lacarra, M., Viegas, O. A., Bilhareus, P., Koetsawang, S., Piya-Anant, M., Diaz, S., Pavez, M., Alvarez, F., Brache, V., LaGuardia, K., Nash, H. and Stern, J. (1997). Levonorgestrel concentrations during use of levonorgestrel rod (LNG ROD) implants. *Contraception,* 55 (2): 81-85.

[10] Reinecke, I., Hofmann, B., Mesic, E., Drenth, H. J. and Garmann, D. (2018). An integrated population pharmacokinetic analysis to characterize levonorgestrel pharmacokinetics after different

administration routes. *The Journal of Clinical Pharmacology,* 58 (12): 1639-1654.

[11] WHO. (2018). *Selected practice recommendations for contraceptive use* [Internet]. WHO. [cited 2018 Sep 18]. Available from: http://www.who.int/reproductivehealth/publications/family_planning/SPR-3/en/.

[12] *Jadelle (Reference ID:4030537). (2016). Highlights of prescribing information.* [cited 2018 Sep 18]. Available from: https://www.accessdata.fda.gov/drugsatfda_docs/label/2016/020544s010lbl.pdf.

[13] Gbolade, B. A. (2010). Failure of Implanon on antituberculous therapy [Internet]. *Open Access Journal of Contraception.* Available from: https://www.dovepress.com/failure-of-implanonreg-on-antituberculous-therapy-peer-reviewed-article-OAJC.

[14] Quest, D. W. (2008). Stockley's drug interactions. 8th edition; Stockley's drug interactions 2008 pocket companion. *Canadian Family Physician,* 54 (7): 1025.

[15] Prevention CDC (C for DC and. U S). (2010). Medical eligibility criteria for contraceptive use, 2010. *MMWR Recomm Rep Morb Mortal Wkly Rep Recomm Rep;* 59(RR-4):1.

[16] Rowlands, S. and Searle, S. (2014). Contraceptive implants: current perspectives. *Open Access Journal of Contraception.* Available from: https://www.dovepress.com/contraceptive-implants-current-perspectives-peer-reviewed-article-OAJC.

In: Obstetric and Gynecology Case Report ISBN: 978-1-53616-711-5
Editor: Dwiana Ocviyanti

Chapter 11

EMBRYO QUALITY AFTER INTRA-CYTOPLASMIC SPERM INJECTION INVOLVING SPERM ASSOCIATED WITH AZOOSPERMIA AND AGED OOCYTES: A CASE REPORT

Silvia W. Lestari[1], Ria Margiana[2] and Achmad Kemal Harzif[3,*]

[1] Department of Medical Biology, Faculty of Medicine, Universitas Indonesia, Jakarta, Indonesia

[2] Department of Anatomy, Faculty of Medicine, Universitas Indonesia, Jakarta, Indonesia

[3]Department of Obstetric and Gynecology, Faculty of Medicine, Universitas Indonesia, Dr. Cipto Mangunkusumo Hospital, Jakarta, Indonesia

Corresponding Author's Email: silvia.lestari@ui.ac.id.

Abstract

Embryo quality determines the pregnancy rate and development of healthy offspring. Embryo profiling can help determine embryo quality through qualification and quantification of various parameters. Here we report a case of successful fertilization with intra-cytoplasmic sperm injection (ICSI) involving sperm associated with azoospermia and aged oocytes. Studies have reported success of ICSI involving sperm associated with azoospermia and aged oocytes, and the findings of the present report will fill the literature gap by providing evidence on the fertilization success rate with ICSI involving sperm associated with azoospermia. A 39-year-old man and 35-year-old woman visited our infertility center. ICSI was performed, and embryos were obtained. Two embryos were freshly transferred on day 3, and two embryos were frozen. As the fresh embryo transfer failed, the frozen embryos were used for frozen embryo transfer, and pregnancy was successfully achieved. We believe that the DNA quality of the testicular sperm determines the pregnancy success rate. Although moderate-quality embryos in frozen embryo transfer were exposed to freezing effects, pregnancy was successfully achieved, possibly because of better receptivity of the endometrium.

Keywords: azoospermia, sperm quality, oocyte quality, sperm retrieval, ICSI, embryo quality

Introduction

The quality of sperm and the transferred embryo are the main determinants of a successful *in vitro* fertilization (IVF) and intra-cytoplasmic sperm injection (ICSI). Although azoospermia, characterized by the absence of viable sperms in the semen, is a major problem, it can be overcome using invasive techniques such as ICSI [1]. Embryo quality should be evaluated because it can help in the identification of embryo markers that can be used to predict the pregnancy rate [2]. Embryo quality provides a more accurate estimate of pregnancy rate compared with the age of the female patient. For creating a successful single-embryo transfer protocol, embryo quality evaluation can be constructive because such an approach will be defined by the results of the embryo quality evaluation [3].

Embryo quality evaluation can also help reduce various risks, such as the risk of multiple gestations in a woman [4]. Similar to oocyte quality assessment, embryo quality assessment can be either invasive or non-invasive [5, 6]. Here we report successful fertilization with ICSI involving sperm associated with azoospermia and aged oocytes. Human embryos have a specific developmental timeline, which determines their morphological features. Embryo quality assessment after ICSI involving sperm associated with azoospermia and aged oocytes provides valuable insights into ICSI and its success rate considering the qualities of the sperms and oocytes.

CASE REPORT

A 39-year-old man and 35-year-old woman visited our infertility center. The man underwent microsurgical epididymal sperm aspiration and testicular sperm aspiration, and the sperms were prepared and selected for ICSI. The woman underwent ovarian stimulation and ovum pick up (OPU), and oocytes were denudated and selected for ICSI.

Ovarian stimulation was performed by the administration of recombinant human follicle-stimulating hormone (FSH) (Gonal-F, Merck Serono, Bari, Italy; 75 IU/ampoule) through daily subcutaneous injections. A gonadotropin-releasing hormone (GnRH) antagonist (Cetrotide 0.25 mg, Merck Serono) was subcutaneously injected when the diameter of the leading follicle was 14–15 mm (Flexible regime); it was continuously administered until the day of human chorionic gonadotropin (hCG) administration. The dose of recombinant human FSH ranged between 150 and 450 IU according to the patient's body mass index, age, and anticipated ovarian response, and it was optimally adjusted depending on the transvaginal ultrasound findings regarding the number and size of growing follicles.

With regard to OPU, hCG was administered when the level of E2 was > 400 pg/mL and two or more follicles reached 17 mm in diameter. Ovulation was induced with 5000–10000 IU hCG (Pregnyl, Merck Serono) or two ampoules (0.1 mg) of triptorelin (Decapeptyl, ___). Oocyte retrieval was performed using an ultrasound-guided needle. The follicles were counted by an embryologist under an inverted microscope and the stages of oocyte maturity were recorded. Before this procedure, denudation of the oocytes was performed. Germinal vesicle and metaphase I oocytes were excluded, and only metaphase II (MII) oocytes were injected in ICSI.

With regard to sperm collection and preparation, the sperm sample was collected on the day of OPU by percutaneous epididymal sperm aspiration (PESA) followed by testicular sperm aspiration (TESA). Both approaches are mainly surgical procedures used to obtain sperm from men with azoospermia for IVF. Sperm preparation involved modified swim-up techniques.

In the ICSI procedure, a single small sperm was directly injected into an oocyte with the aim of increasing the probability of success with IVF. The micromanipulation techniques were performed using an IVF laboratory micromanipulator [4]. The sperm was suctioned using an injecting pipette and was then infiltrated into the ooplasm at the 3-o′clock position. Injected oocytes were placed in a culture dish. The fertilized oocytes were observed for both growth and development. Selected embryos were later transferred to the uterus [7].

Table 1. Embryo grading [8]

Measurement	Grade	Description
	Grade 1	Embryo with blastomeres of equal size, no cytoplasmic fragments
	Grade 2	Embryo with blastomeres of equal size, minor cytoplasmic fragments
Cleavage stage morphology	Grade 3	Embryo with blastomeres of distinctly of unequal size, none or few cytoplasmic fragments
	Grade 4	Embryo with blastomeres of equal or unequal size, significant cytoplasmic fragments
	Grade 5	Embryo with few blastomeres of any size, severe or complete fragments

In embryo culture, each embryo was individually evaluated under a microscope early in the morning from day 1 to day 3. Embryo grading is presented in Table 1. The fertilization rate was defined as the ratio of the number of two-pronuclear (2PN) zygotes to the number of injected MII oocytes (fertilization rate = [number of 2PN zygotes on the 1st day]/[total number of injected oocytes] × 100).

The embryos are presented in Figure 1. Embryos that were selected for transfer were incubated in a transfer dish until they were loaded in a transfer catheter on the day of transfer. Four embryos were used. Embryos A and B were transferred freshly on day 3, and the other two embryos (embryos C and D) were frozen. As the fresh embryo transfer failed, the frozen embryos were used in frozen embryo transfer.

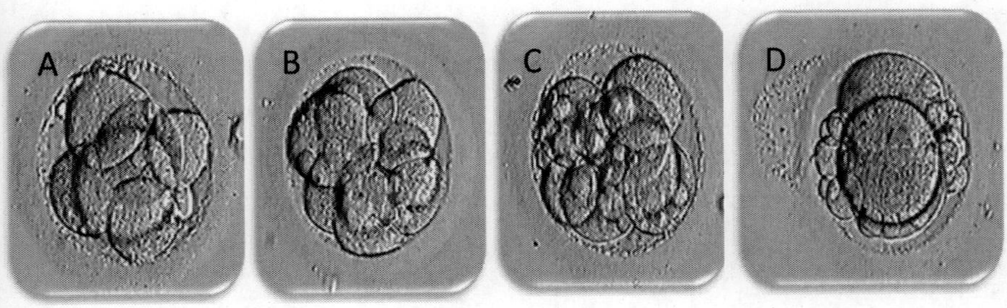

Figure 1. Embryos on day 3. (A) Eight-cell embryo; (B) Six-cell embryo; (C) Six-cell embryo + fragments; (D) Three-cell embryo + fragments.

DISCUSSION

The present report is important, as the reproduction potential of men with azoospermia is not clear. In the woman, a GnRH antagonist protocol (n = 73) was initiated in addition to recombinant human FSH administration (75 IU/ampoule t.d.i) by subcutaneous injection until the day of hCG administration. Then, ovulation was induced followed by oocyte retrieval and denudation and eventually sperm injection. Women between the ages of 35 and 40 years have 14.2 ± 7.1 reductions in oocytes, and this is associated with a 16% reduction in the pregnancy rate among these women [9]. If the number of grade A embryos is greater than five, the pregnancy rate is not affected [10]. Advancing age can affect the pregnancy rate and the number of good-quality embryos. If an aged woman can produce a high number of good-quality embryos, the pregnancy rate is not affected. Azoospermia can only reduce the chance of fertilization but cannot prevent fertilization if ICSI can be performed.

Embryo quality evaluation involving invasive techniques, such as ICSI, is common in human assisted reproductive technology. Fertilization might be unsuccessful because of poor quality of either the sperm or oocyte. Sperm from men with azoospermia can successfully fertilize an oocyte through ICSI. Our male patient had obstructive azoospermia, and the obtained sperm successfully fertilized oocytes. This is consistent with the finding of Esteves that the fertilization rate and embryo implantation rate were significantly lower in non-obstructive azoospermia than in obstructive azoospermia [11].

In the present case, sperms were retrieved from the testis, as retrieval from the epididymis failed. Although the sperm in the epididymis undergo a maturation process and differ from sperm in the testis, the obtained sperm successfully fertilized oocytes. This is consistent with the finding of Silber that there was no difference in outcomes between fresh epididymis sperm and testicular sperm [12].

Oocytes are affected by age, and aged oocytes reduce the chances of successful fertilization [17]. The number of healthy oocytes tends to reduce with age [4]. In this case report, the fertilization rate was 41.7%, while the morphological embryo grade raged from grade 2 to 4. This confirmed the finding of Cimadomo et al. [1] that aged oocytes were associated with chromosome abnormalities, such as premature separation of sister chromatid and reverse segregation [13], and that the reduced female reproductive capacity with age was associated with gradual depletion of oocytes from the ovary and a decrease in oocyte quality [3, 6, 14].

In this report, although moderate-quality embryos (grades 2–4) in frozen embryo transfer had already been exposed to the cryoprotectant and freezing effects, pregnancy was successful. On the other hand, fresh embryo transfer was not successful. This might be because of good receptivity in frozen embryo transfer that could not be achieved in fresh embryo transfer [15].

This is consistent with the finding of Wintner et al. [16] that a poor-quality embryo did not affect a good-quality embryo when transferred together in a negative condition.

CONCLUSION

Clinical pregnancy was successfully achieved, possibly because of the better DNA quality of the testicular sperm compared with that of the aged oocytes. Although moderate-quality embryos in frozen embryo transfer were exposed to freezing effects, pregnancy was successfully achieved, possibly because of better receptivity of the endometrium.

ACKNOWLEDGMENT

The authors sincerely thank the Director of Anna Hospital, Bekasi, and Chief of SMART IVF Anna Hospital for their permission and clinical assistance during the patient's management.

REFERENCES

[1] Cimadomo, D., Fabozzi, G., Vaiarelli, A., Ubaldi, N., Ubaldi, F.M., Rienzi, L. (2018). Impact of maternal age on oocyte and embryo competence. *Front. Endocrinol*, 9 : 327.

[2] Kanto, S., Arai, Y., Kyono, K. (2008). Fresh Motile testicular sperm retrieved from non- obstructive azoospermic patients has the same potential to achieve fertilization and pregnancy via icsi as sperm retrieved from obstructive azoospermic patients. *J. Urol*, 179 : 593.

[3] Ahmed, M., Shareef, O., Adam, I., Rayis, D. (2015). Maternal age and intracytoplasmic sperm injection outcome in infertile couples at Khartoum, Sudan. *F1000Res*, 4 : 1339.

[4] Herrero, B., Lusignan, M., Son, W., Buckett, W., Chan, P. (2016). Effects of sperm quality on the success of intracytoplasmic sperm injection (ICSI) with testicular sperm in couples with recurrent ICSI failure with ejaculated sperm. *Fertil. Steril*, 106 :e226.

[5] Loutradis, D., Drakakis, P., Kallianidis, K., Milingos, S., Dendrinos, S., Michalas, S. (1999). Oocyte morphology correlates with embryo quality and pregnancy rate after intracytoplasmic sperm injection. *Fertil. Steril*, 72 : 240-244.

[6] Ge, Z., Schatten, H., Zhang, C., Sun, Q. (2015). Oocyte aging and epigenetics. *Reproduction,* 149: R103-R114.

[7] Gunby, J., Daya, S., IVF Directors Group of the Canadian Fertility and Andrology Society, (2005). Assisted reproductive technologies (ART) in Canada: 2001 results from the Canadian ART Register. *Fertil. Steril,* 84 :590-599.

[8] Veeck, L.L. (1988). Oocyte assessment and biological performance. *Ann. NY Acad*, 541 :259-274.

[9] Zegers-Hochschild, F., Nygren, K.G., Adamson, G.D., de Mouzon, J., Lancaster, P., Mansour, R., Sullivan, E., International Committee Monitoring Assisted Reproductive Technologies, (2006). The International Committee Monitoring Assisted Reproductive Technologies (ICMART) glossary on ART terminology. *Fertil. Steril*, 86 : 16-19.

[10] Yu, Y., Xu, Q., Pan, Y., Jiang, Y., Zhang, H., Li, L., Liu, R. (2018). Pregnancy and neonatal outcomes in azoospermic men after intracytoplasmic sperm injection using testicular sperm and donor sperm. *Med. Sci. Monit,* 24 : 6968-6974.

[11] Esteves, S.C. (2015). Clinical management of infertile men with non-obstructive azoospermia. *Asian J. Androl*,17 :459-470.

[12] Silber, S.J. (1995) Epididymal and testicular spermatozoa and intracytoplasmic sperm injection. *Assist. Reprod. Rev*, 6 : 45-53.

[13] Grøndahl, M.L., Christiansen, S.L., Kesmodel, U.S., Agerholm, I.E., Lemmen, J.G., Lundstrøm, P. (2017). Effect of women's age on embryo morphology, cleavage rate and competence-A multicenter cohort study. *PLoS One,* 12 :12.

[14] Babayev, E., Seli, E. (2015). Oocyte mitochondrial function and reproduction. *Curr. Opin. Obstet. Gynecol,* 27 :175-181.

[15] Bancroft, J. (2009). Sexual aspects of fertility, fertility control and infertility. In: *Human Sexuality and Its Problems*, 3rd edition : 439-463).

[16] Wintner, E.M., Klement, A.H., Tzadikevitch, K., Ghetler, Y., Gonen, O., Wintner, O., Shulman, A., Wiser, A. (2017). Does the transfer of a poor quality embryo together with a good quality embryo affect the In Vitro Fertilization (IVF) outcome? *J. Ovarian Res*, 10 : 2.

In: Obstetric and Gynecology Case Report
Editor: Dwiana Ocviyanti
ISBN: 978-1-53616-711-5

Chapter 12

ROLE OF PREIMPLANTATION GENETIC SCREENING IN A CASE OF RECURRENT *IN VITRO* FERTILIZATION FAILURE

Budi Wiweko[1], Riyan Hari Kurniawan[2], Pritta Iffanolida[3], Kresna Mutia[3], Gita Pratama[1], Kanadi Sumapraja[1], Achmad Kemal Harzif[1], Muharam Natadisastra[1] and Andon Hestiantoro[1,*]

[1]Division of Reproductive Endocrinology and Infertility,
Department of Obstetrics and Gynecology,
Faculty of Medicine, Universitas Indonesia,
Dr. Cipto Mangunkusumo Hospital, Jakarta, Indonesia
[2]Division of Health Reproduction,
Department of Obstetrics and Gynecology, Faculty of Medicine,
Universitas Indonesia, Dr. Cipto Mangunkusumo Hospital,
Jakarta, Indonesia

[*] Corresponding Author's E-mail: hestiantoro@gmail.com.

[3]Indonesian Reproductive Medicine Research and Training Center (INA-REPROMED) of Faculty of Medicine, Universitas Indonesia, Dr. Cipto Mangunkusumo Hospital, Jakarta, Indonesia

ABSTRACT

In-vitro fertilization (IVF) is a process by which egg is fertilized by sperm outside the body or coined as in-vitro. IVF is the most clearly indicated when infertility results from one or more causes having no other effective treatment and often be the best treatment for couples with multifactor infertility because it can address or overcome all contributing causes at the same time. Concurrent with an IVF cycle, it is possible to obtain a cellular biopsy from a developing embryo and genetically evaluate this sample such as preimplantation genetic screening (PGS). PGS is the practice to evaluate embryos for chromosomal aneuploidy. Mrs. BJP, a 38-year-old female, came to the hospital with recurrent IVF failure. She had a history of two attempts of intrauterine insemination (IUI) and a history of three IVF attempts but has not been impregnanted. Physical examination revealed BMI 20.4kg/m^2 and gynecologic status within normal limit. Transvaginal ultrasound examination revealed that uterus position ante flexion, size and shape within normal limit, endometrium regular 9mm, both ovaries in normal size. Ovarian stimulation used total rFSH 3300 IU. Oocyte retrieval was performed and got 7 oocytes, 3 were fertilized, and then 2 embryos were frozen. We performed PGS to both embryos and the results were one embryo normal and one embryo aneuploidy.

We performed single embryo transfer and patient succeeded in getting pregnant. Morphologically normal looking embryos can still harbor genetic or epigenetic defect. The objective of IVF is to place the single best embryo. It is important to consider the method of embryo selection.

Keywords: subfertility, IVF failure, PGS, single embryo transfer

INTRODUCTION

In-vitro fertilization (IVF) is a process by which egg is fertilized by sperm outside the body or coined as in-vitro. IVF is the advanced clinical treatment for infertility.

IVF is the most clearly indicated when infertility results from one or more causes having no other effective treatment; severe tubal disease relating to previous infection or advanced endometriosis and severe male factor infertility are the most obvious examples. IVF also is often the best treatment for couples with multifactor infertility because it can address or overcome all contributing causes at the same time. IVF is a legitimate treatment option for women with age-related or otherwise unexplained infertility and represents the treatment of last resort when other treatments fail.

Concurrent with an IVF cycle, it is possible to obtain a cellular biopsy from a developing embryo and genetically evaluate this sample [1]. Preimplantation genetic screening (PGS) is the practice to evaluate embryos for chromosomal aneuploidy, the presence of either too few or too many chromosomes, in chromosomally normal parents. Meanwhile, preimplantation genetics diagnosis (PGD) is the practice of evaluating embryos for specific genetic abnormalities, such as cystic fibrosis, where carrier status has been documented in each of the parents and sickle cell disease [1].

CASE REPORT

Mrs. BJP, a 38-year-old female, came to the hospital with recurrent IVF failure. She had been having secondary subfertility for 7 years and had a history of cesarean section, without history of contraception use. She had regular menstruation (28 days). In 2013, she had a history of two attempts of intrauterine insemination (IUI) in Jakarta but did not get pregnant. In 2013 and 2018, she had three attempts pf IVF in Malaysia but still did not get pregnant.

Physical examination revealed a body mass index of 20.4kg/m^2, and gyne-cological findings were normal. Transvaginal ultrasound examination revealed that the uterus was in anteflexion, with a normal size and shape (Figure 1), the endometrium was regular at 9mm, and both ovaries had normal sizes (Figure 2).

She received ovarian stimulation with a total recombinant follicle-stimulating hormone dose of 3300 IU. Oocyte retrieval was performed, and seven oocytes were obtained. Eventually, three were fertilized and two embryos were frozen.

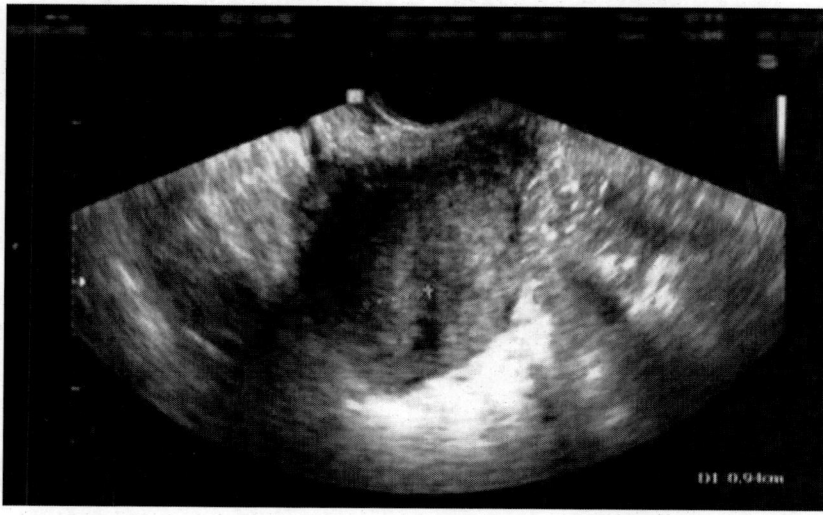

Figure 1. Ultrasound of the uterus.

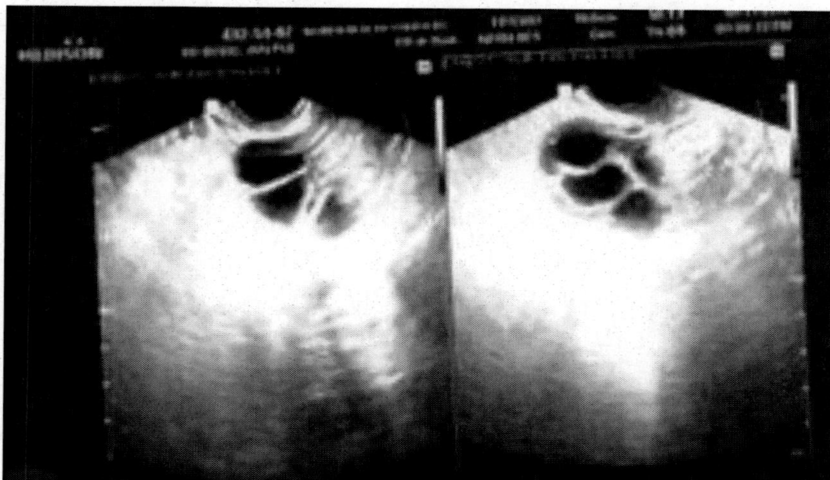

Figure 2. Ultrasound of the ovaries.

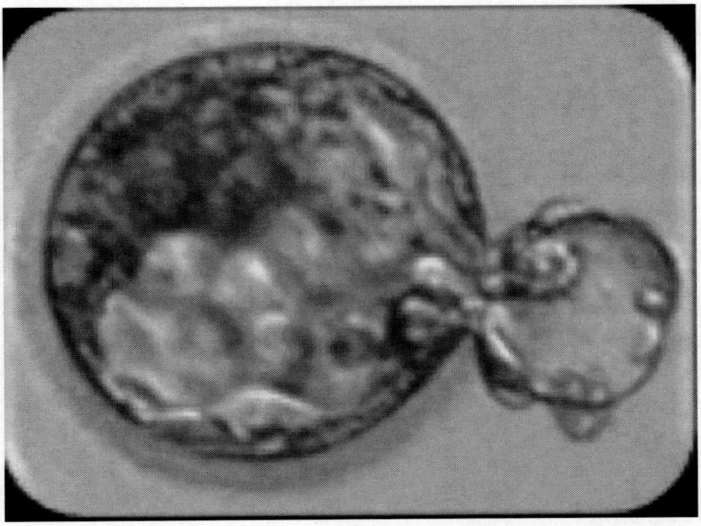

Figure 3. Embryo 1 without chromosomal abnormality.

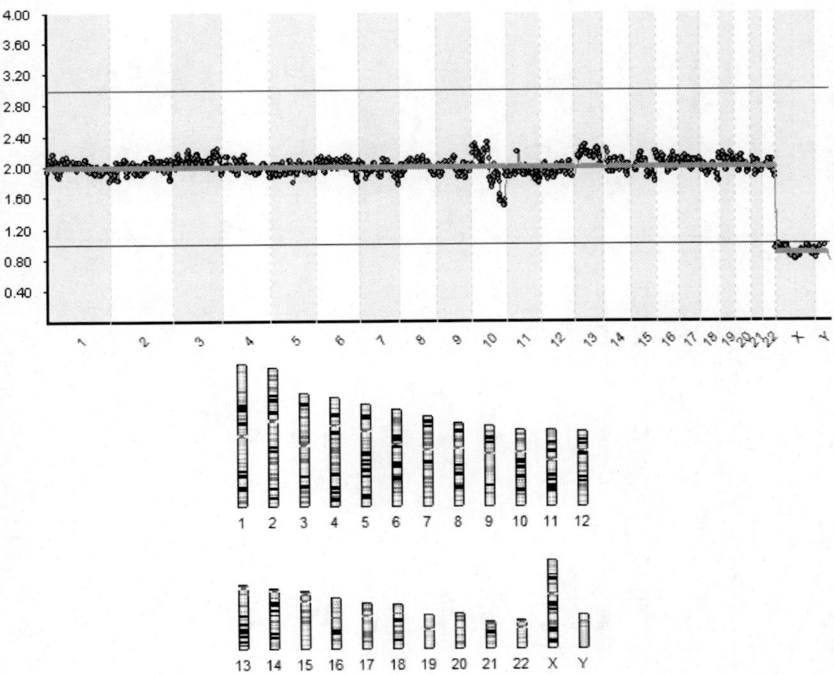

Figure 4. Next-generation sequencing of embryo 1. There is no chromosomal Abnormality.

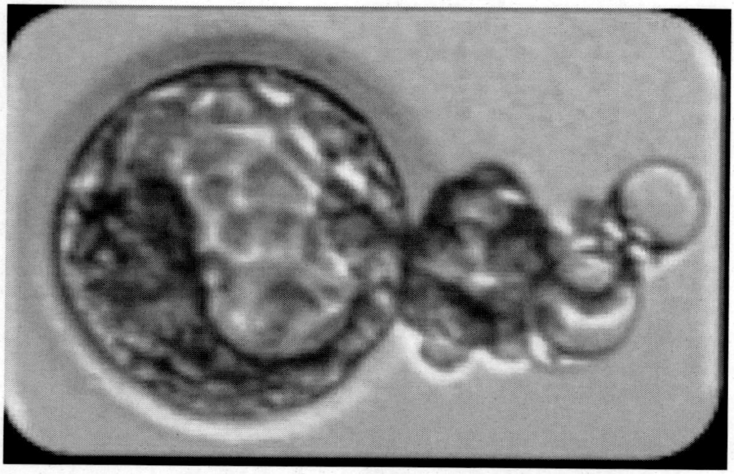

Figure 5. Embryo 2 with chromosomal abnormality.

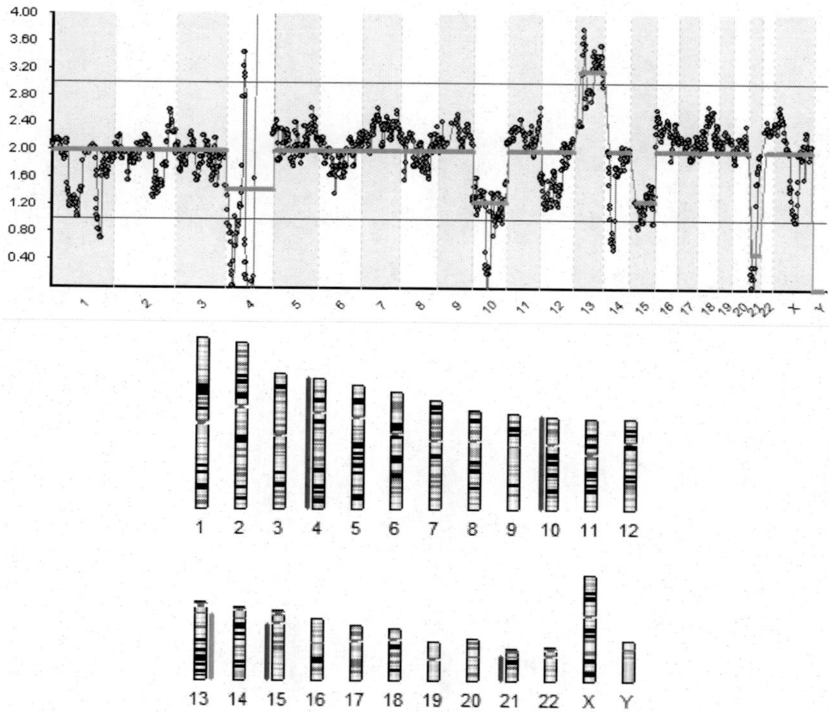

Figure 6. Next-generation sequencing of embryo 2. There is chromosomal abnormality.

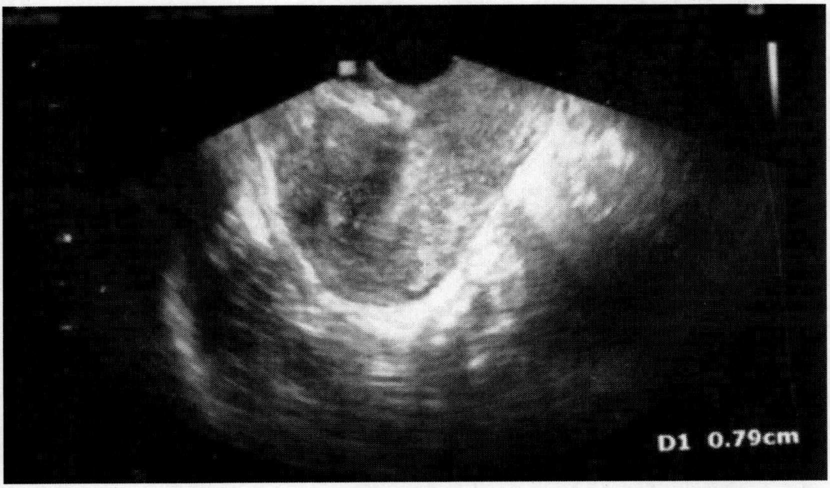

Figure 7. Gestational sac (intrauterine).

PGS was performed in both embryos, and it was found that one embryo was normal (Figures 3 and 4) and one embryo had aneuploidy (Figures 5 and 6).

Single embryo transfer was performed, and she successfully became pregnant, with βhCG 1783mIU/mL and progesterone 9.39ng/mL (Figure 7).

DISCUSSION

Preimplantation genetic screening describes testing for oocyte or embryo aneuploidy when the parents are known or presumed to be normal. Indication of PGS includes older women, history of PRL, repeated IVF failure and severe male factor infertility.

The concept of PGS suggests that by determining embryo ploidy in human embryos prior to embryo transfer, IVF outcomes will be improved because transfers of aneuploid embryos are avoided [2].

Preimplantation genetic testing (PGT) broadly describes procedures involving the removal of one or more nuclei from polar bodies (oocytes) or cells (blastomeres, trophoectoderm) from embryos to test for mutations or evaluate their chromosomal complement. Preimplantation genetic diagnosis (PGD) describes testing for a known genetic abnormality carried by one or both parents to determine whether it has been transmitted to the oocyte or embryo.

PGD is no longer considered experimental, and implementation of newly developed methods for genetic analysis will likely continue to broaden its application [3].

PGS has no effect on perinatal outcomes among women experiencing recurrent IVF failure [4, 5]. Results of this genetic analysis direct to choose the embryos for uterine transfer. PGS can only be performed using cells obtained at embryo biopsy, this technology is only possible in conjunction with an IVF cycle [1].

Selecting chromosomally normal embryos for replacement should increase implantation rates, reduce spontaneous miscarriage rates, reduce aneuploid conceptions, and improve delivery rates in assisted reproductive technology cycles [6, 9]. The number referrals for PGS has only increased since its first clinical application [10].

In this case, the patient was performed frozen embryo transfer with single euploid blastocyst transfer. The result after 2 weeks after frozen embryo transfer showed intrauterin GS, βhCG 1783mIU/mL and progesterone 9.39ng/mL.

Single embryo transfer can reduce multiple pregnancies which is achieved from multiple embryos that were transferred after an IVF. Multiple pregnancies that is known to cause adverse maternal and fetal outcomes [4].

Single blastocyst transfer is an effective method to reduce the risk of multiple births without compromising the pregnancy outcomes [4].

CONCLUSION

Morphologically normal-looking embryos can still harbor genetic or epigenetic defect. The objective of IVF is to place single best embryo. It is important to consider the method of embryo selection.

Defining the exact benefit conferred by PGS and determining exactly which patient populations could be best served by PGS, however, is currently controversial.

In the near future, several large and high quality studies will attempt to answer these questions. PGS is increasingly being applied to patients with ever-expanding clinical indications.

References

[1] Brezina, P. R., Ke, R. W., Kutteh, W. H. (2013). Preimplantation Genetic Screening: A Practical Guide. *Clin. Med. Insights Reprod. Health,* 7 : 37 - 42.

[2] Orvieto, R., Gleicher, N., (2016). Should preimplantation genetic screening (pgs) be implemented to routine IVF practice? *J. Assist. Reprod. Genet.,* 33 : 1445 - 1448.

[3] Society or Assisted Reproductive Technology. (2008). American Society or Reproductive Medicine: Preimplantation genetic testing: a Practice Committee opinion. *Fertil. Steril.,* 90: S136.

[4] Sundhararaj, U. M., Madne, M. V., Bliangady, R., Gurunath, S., Swamy, A. G., Gopal, I. S. (2017). Single blastocyst transfer: the key to reduce multiple pregnancy rates without compromising the live birth rate. *J. Hum. Reprod. Sci.,* 10 : 201 - 207.

[5] Hatirnaz, S., Ozer, A., Hatirnaz, E., Atasever, M., Başaranoglu, S., Kanat-Pektas, M., Api, M. (2017). Pre-implantation genetic screening among women experiencing recurrent failure of in vitro fertilization. *Int. J. Gynaecol. Obstet.,* 137 : 314 - 318.

[6] Platteau, P., Staessen, C., Michiels, A., Tournaye, H., Van Steirteghem, A., Liebaers, I. and Devroey, P. (2004). Comparison of the aneuploidy frequency in embryos derived from testicular sperm extraction in obstructive and non-obstructive azoospermic men. *Hum. Reprod.,* 19 : 1570 - 1574.

[7] Donoso, P., Platteau, P., Papanikolaou, E. G., Staessen, C., Van Steirteghem, A., Devroey, P. (2006). Does PGD for aneuploidy

screening change the selection of embryos derived from testicular sperm extraction in obstructive and non-obstructive azoospermic men? *Hum. Reprod.,* 21: 2390 - 2395.

[8] Gianaroli, L., Magli, M. C., Ferraretti, A. P., Munne, S. (1999). Preimplantation diagnosis for aneuploidies in patients undergoing in vitro fertilization with a poor prognosis: identification of the categories for which it should be proposed. *Fertil. Steril.,* 72 : 837 - 844.

[9] Munne, S., Magli, C., Cohen, J., Morton, P., Sadowy, S., Gianaroli, L., Tucker, M., Márquez, C., Sable, D., Ferraretti, A. P., Massey, J. B. (1999). Positive outcome after preimplantation diagnosis of aneuploidy in human embryos. *Hum. Reprod.,* 14 : 2191 - 2199.

[10] Verlinsky, Y., Cieslak, J., Freidine, M., Lvakhnenko, V., Wolf, G., Kovalinskaya, L., White, M., Lifchez, A., Kaplan, B., Moise, J., Valle, J. (1995). Pregnancies following preconceptiondiagnosis of common aneuploidies by fluorescent in-situhybridization. *Hum. Reprod.,* 10 : 1923 - 1927.

In: Obstetric and Gynecology Case Report ISBN: 978-1-53616-711-5
Editor: Dwiana Ocviyanti

Chapter 13

Bio-Psychosocial Aspects of Infertility: Illustrative Case of Recurrent Failure with Assisted Reproductive Technologies

***Hari Sandi Sumardi*[1,*] *and Dwiana Ocviyanti*[2]**

[1]Faculty of Medicine, Universitas Indonesia, Jakarta, Indonesia

[2]Department of Obstetric and Gynecology, Faculty of Medicine, Universitas Indonesia, Dr. Cipto Mangunkusumo Hospital, Jakarta, Indonesia

Abstract

Infertility is associated with psychological problems being experienced by both partners, and *in vitro* fertilization (IVF) is one of many infertility treatment procedures. IVF significantly influences patients and their family's psychology. This report reviews the biopsychosocial aspectsof infertility in relation to recurrent IVF failure. A 42-year-old

---

* Corresponding Author's Email: harysandidr@gmail.com.

female patient with primary infertility for the past 16 years requested consultation on pregnancy programs. She had a history of cystectomy surgery for endometriotic cysts. At presentation, there were no problems with the husband's sperm quality, the patient had undergone three failed insemination attempts, followed by three failed IVF attempts. Ultrasound examination found left tubal enlargement size $25 \times 13 \times 16$ mm^3, correspond to hydrosalpinx. The patient was also diagnosed as having diminished ovarian reserves. She underwent a hysteroscopy with subsequent laparoscopy for endometriosis in the left fallopian tube, which resulted in a left-sided salpingectomy. After laparoscopic surgery, the patient plans to undergo one final IVF procedure. After failed IVF cycles, women experience an increase in depressive symptoms with lower levels of self-esteem, compared to those before the treatment cycle. A problem-solving coping strategy is associated with better psychological adjustment, whereas the use of avoidance coping and social isolation has the opposite effect; hence, behavioral strategies may help these patients deal with their loss of control. In conclusion. This case illustrates the association between infertility and ART failure and its biopsychosocial implications that require appropriate support to reduce patient distress, help patients come to terms with their situation, and facilitate decision making.

Keywords: assisted reproduction, unsuccessful IVF treatment, stress, treatment failure

INTRODUCTION

Infertility is defined as the inability to conceive after 1 year of unprotected intercourse of reasonable frequency [1], and it is a serious concern that affects about one in 10 couples [3]. It may affect the relationship between the couple, their families, or friends, as well as decrease their self-confidence because of feelings of guilt and insufficiency [4]. Furthermore, procedures used for the diagnosis and treatment of infertility can affect both partners and regrettably lead to emotional stress and a reduction in the quality of life (QoL) [5]. Previously published psychosocial studies reveal a greater prevalence of negative attitudes in infertile individuals, such as dissatisfaction, unwillingness, and disorientation regarding treatment [6]. Therefore, it is extremely important to evaluate the psychosocial background of the couple undergoing treatment to minimize distracting factors and to sustain patient compliance with treatment.

Assisted reproductive technologies (ARTs) are a well-established [7] and important treatment option for those seeking help for conception [2]. However, despite advances in ARTs and an increase in their use [6], the success rate of ART, conventionally defined as the rate of live births per cycle initiated [8] remains modest [9].

Couples who want descent through an ART program have high hopes of achieving success, on the contrary it can cause disappointment if this program fails [10]. A systematic review of psychological adjustments to ART found that, overall, women were able to adjust well to the unsuccessful treatment cycle [11]. Similarly from other studies concluded that there were no changes in emotions and that there were positive emotional adjustments after experiencing treatment failure [12]. But on the contrary, many other studies have reported that women and men experience negative psychological effects after unsuccessful ART [13]. With the increasing number of couples who want ART treatment, including couples with old age, it is important to assess all the potential psychological effects associated with treatment failure and also consider wisely about funding, access and feasibility. This report discusses the biopsychosocial aspects of infertility by describing an illustrative case with recurrent ART failure.

CASE ILLUSTRATION

A 42-year-old female patient presented to the RSCM Endocrinology polyclinic for consultation on pregnancy programs. Married in 2002, she had a 16-year history of primary infertility. The couple began to undergo treatment for infertility in 2007. However, she had to undergo a cystectomy in the same year for endometriotic cysts. After she received this surgery, the husband underwent treatment with urologists for increasing the sperm quality. However, the couple did not continue with the follow-up treatment. In 2015, the couple attempted insemination thrice at another hospital. As all three inseminations had failed, they subsequently received IVF treatment three times, twice in another hospital in 2017 and once atour facility in 2018. Unfortunately, all three IVF cycles were unsuccessful. Currently, the patient has regular menstruationand does nothave symptoms of dysmenorrhea, dyspareunia, dyschezia, or dysuria.

A general physical examination anda gynecological examination were unremarkable. Hysterosalpingogram (HSG) examination revealed that the right fallopian tube was patent, but the left tube was non-patent.

Uterine ultrasound revealed a 38-mm endometrium line and a negative triple line, along with a non-homogenous myometrium with a hyper-echoic mass of indistinguishable tissue of the size 24 × 30 × 18 mm. Several smaller sized (<10 mm) masses were also present, but without an intra cavitary mass. The endocervix was normal, the right ovary showed a follicular diameter of 12 mm, and the left ovary did not appear to have a follicle. In addition, left tubal enlargement was found with a25 × 13 × 16 mm hydrosalpinx. These findings led to the diagnosis ofdiminished ovarian reserves, a three-time history of IVF failure, primary infertility for the past 16 years, and left hydrosalpinx.

The patient subsequently underwent laparoscopic cystectomy. Hysteroscopy revealed a normal-portioned uterus, normal endocervix, uterine cavity within a normal range, a closed left tubal ostium, and an open right tubal ostium. Furthermore, the laparoscopy revealed adhesion to the omentum, specifically, a3-cm left adnexal mass attached to the sigmoid, for which adhesiolysis was performed, which released a brown fluid, consistent with endometriosis. A left salpingectomy was performed based on the above findings. The patient plans to undergo another IVF procedure after recovering from the surgery.

Discussion

As infertility includes medical, psychological, and social problems, a biopsychosocial model wasused to address the dynamic relationship between the biological, psychological, and social aspects of infertility. All these aspects are crucial as they influence our understanding and treatment of the infertile couple. The biopsychosocial model may also be used to address collaborative or multidisciplinary approaches to care for an infertile couple.

Biological Aspects

Biological effects refer to the effects of infertility, including multiple medical diagnoses, causes of infertility, and medical interventions. Empirical data provide an estimate of the primary causes of infertility: female factors, accounting approximately to 35%–45%; male factors, accounting to 35%–40%; combined factors, accounting to 15%–20%; and residual factors for which no explanation can be determined using current diagnostic methods, accounting to 10%–15%. Specific causes can only be determined by an extensive workup, which typically includesmultiple physical examinations, frequent review of basal body temperature, intercourse records, laboratory tests, radiologic tests, surgery, and trials of medical treatment.

Psychological Aspects

Infertility and its treatments have a significant impact on a person's QoL. For instance, infertility isnegatively associated with relational, sexual, and psychosocial well-being. Patients with infertility also experience increased stress and tensionin the relationship with their partner. Although not all individuals perceive infertility as a crisis, research indicates that infertility can be a difficult and painful grieving process for the infertile couple [5].

Infertility is not just a medical condition to be treated using fertility drugs, surgeries, or ARTs. Rather, it is often a crisis that profoundly affects nearly all aspects of the patient's personality and life [5]. Therefore, best practices in fertility care should include a holistic approach that considers QoL as integral to the clinical practice. QoL comprises domains such as emotional well-being, social functioning, physical health, patient environment, and personal beliefs, and can be assessed using both generic and condition-specific instruments.

A study by Menning et al. in the 1980s reported that infertile couples require psychological support. The Fertility Quality of Life Questionnaire, which is an international and condition-specific tool that realistically evaluates the effects of infertility on the QoL, can reveal the psychometric characteristics of individuals with greater objectivity [14].

Social Aspects

The social component of infertility must be evaluated in social structures and social organizations such as family and society. In families, girls are usually taught that being a mother is the highest expression of womanhood. From a communal perspective, families ensure that current and old members of society will be replaced regularly when there is a new generation Thus, there are societal constraints and messages that direct how infertile individuals and couples deal with childlessness [6].

Women more than men, who are infertile, tend to ask themselves who they are if they cannot become a parent, and thereby make infertility a definition of their self rather than a medical condition. As their infertility becomes more undeniable, there is a great sense of isolation from others during social discussions of pregnancy, childbirth, and childrearing [15].

Biopsychosocial Aspects of ART

For the couple described in the illustrative case, the best opportunity for evaluation and treatment lies within the domain of ARTs. Other alternatives include adoption and surrogate motherhood [6].

Factors associated with lower success rates for ART include duration of infertility, greater number of ART cycles, and increasing maternal age [12]. With increasing maternal age, the live delivery rate per thawed embryo declines, and this is similar tousing autologous fresh embryos [13]. Internationally, women aged 40 yearsor more are increasingly undergoing ART [16].

The impact of failure of ART on individual psychosocial conditions is not taken into consideration when assessing the safety and effectiveness of treatment, nor is it included in the assessment aspect in making decisions about the direction of decisions in choosing ART treatment (17). Conversely, the potential for psychosocial gains through the success of ART, or even through ART efforts is more widely delivered. ART clinicians only always convey more of the impact of positive psychological aspects in undergoing this treatment than to expose more of the adverse psychological effects associated with failure of ART therapy (18).

After a failed IVF cycle, women experience an increase in depressive symptoms and lower levels of self-esteem, compared to those before the treatment cycle. A problem-solving coping strategy has been associated with better psychological adjustment, whereas the use of avoidance coping and social isolation has the opposite effect. Hence, behavioral strategies may help these patients deal with their perceived loss of control [6].

A meta-analysis to determine the association between depression and anxiety and ART treatment outcomes reported that both depression and anxiety increased after ART treatment failure. In contrast, depression decreased after a successful treatment cycle, and both depression and anxiety decreased with time. Nonetheless, these feelings remained higher than baselline measure in the group with the failed outcome even six months after the prosedur. Studies included in the narrative synthesis also confirmed an association with negative psychological outcomes in relation to marital satisfaction and general well-being following treatment failure.

Conclusion

More than in any other area of obstetrics and gynecology, infertility carefor a partner with recurrent IVF failureinvolves biopsychosocial aspects that require appropriate support to reduce patient distress, help the patient to come to terms with her situation, and facilitate decision making. Training aimed at recognizing and managing these biopsychosocial aspects of infertility and assisted reproduction should be a part of the training requirements for generalists and subspecialists, and such training should include psychosexual counseling, the role of cognitive behavioral therapy, issues relating to same-sex partnerships, single parenthood, gender identity, gamete preservation, and surrogate motherhood. Clinicians should be prepared to confront and address these issues using a patient-centered holistic approach not only during all interactions and at each step of the investigation and treatment process, but also through referrals to tailored counseling services in specific situations that require a trained mental health professional.

REFERENCES

[1] Hoffman, B. L., Schorge J. O,. Bradshaw, K.D., Halvorson, L.M., Schaffer J.I., Corton M. M. (2016). *Williams gynecology*. New York: McGraw-Hill.

[2] Karaca, N., Karabulut, A., Ozkan, S., Aktun, H., Orengul, F., Yilmaz, R., et al. (2016). Effect of IVF failure on quality of life and emotional status in infertile couples. *European Journal of Obstetrics & Gynecology and Reproductive Biology*, 206:158–63.

[3] Boivin, J., Takefman, J., Braverman, A. (2011). The fertility quality of life (FertiQoL) tool: development and general psychometric properties†. *Human Reproduction*, 26(8): 2084–91.

[4] Milazzo, A., Mnatzaganian, G., Elshaug, A. G, Hemphill, S. A., Hiller, J. E., on behalf of The Astute Health Study Group. (2016). Depression and Anxiety Outcomes Associated with Failed Assisted Reproductive Technologies: A Systematic Review and Meta-Analysis. Lambalk CB, editor. *PLOS ONE*, 11(11): e0165805.

[5] Aarts, J. W. M., van Empel, I. W. H., Boivin, J., Nelen, W. L., Kremer, J. A. M., Verhaak, C. M. (2011). Relationship between quality of life

and distress in infertility: a validation study of the Dutch FertiQoL. *Human Reproduction,* 26(5):1112–8.

[6] Grinion, P. E., (2005). The biopsychosocial stress of infertility: grappling with the ethical and moral concerns VIS-À-VIS Assisted Reproductive Technologies. NACSW Convention.

[7] Zegers-Hochschild F., Adamson, G. D., de Mouzon, J., Ishihara, O., Mansour, R., Nygren, K, et al. (2009). International Committee for Monitoring Assisted Reproductive Technology (ICMART) and the World Health Organization (WHO) revised glossary of ART terminology.*Fertility and Sterility*, 92(5):1520–4.

[8] Heredia, M., Tenías, J. M., Rocio, R., Amparo, F., Calleja, M. A., Valenzuela, J. C., (2013). Quality of life and predictive factors in patients undergoing assisted reproduction techniques. *European Journal of Obstetrics & Gynecology and Reproductive Biology*,167(2):176–80.

[9] Domar, A.D., Broome, A., Zuttermeister, P. C., Seibel, M., Friedman, R. (1992). The prevalence and predictability of depression in infertile women **Supported by grant 5R03MH45591 from the National Institute of Mental Health, Bethesda, Maryland.††Presented at the Annual Meeting of The American Fertility Society, Orlando, Florida, October 21 to 24, 1991. *Fertility and Sterility*. 58(6):1158–63.

[10] Gourounti, K., Anagnostopoulos, F., Potamianos, G., Lykeridou, K., Schmidt, L., Vaslamatzis, G. (2012). Perception of control, coping and psychological stress of infertile women undergoing IVF. *Reproductive BioMedicine Online*, 24(6):670–9.

[11] Verhaak, C. M., Smeenk, J. M. J., Evers, A. W. M., Kremer, J. A. M., Kraaimaat, F. W., Braat, D. D. M. (2007). Women's emotional adjustment to IVF: a systematic review of 25 years of research. *Human Reproduction Update*. 13(1):27–36.

[12] Karabulut, A., Özkan, S., Oğuz, N. (2013.). Predictors of fertility quality of life (FertiQoL) in infertile women: analysis of confounding factors. *European Journal of Obstetrics & Gynecology and Reproductive Biology*,170(1):193–7.

[13] Chachamovich, J., Chachamovich, E., Fleck, M. P,, Cordova, F. P., Knauth, D., Passos, E. (2009). Congruence of quality of life among infertile men and women: findings from a couple-based study. *Human Reproduction.* 24(9):2151–7.

[14] Maroufizadeh, S., Ghaheri, A., Amini, P., Samani, R. O. (2017). Psychometric Properties of The Fertility Quality of Life Instrument in Infertile Iranian Women. *Int J Fertil Steril*, 10(4): 371-79.

[15] Fisher, J. R., Hammarberg, K. (2012). Psychological and social aspects of infertility in men: an overview of the evidence and implications for psychologically informed clinical care and future research. *Asian Journal of Andrology,* 14(1):121–9.

[16] Noorbala, A. A., Ramazanzadeh, F., Malekafzali, H., Abedinia, N., Forooshani, A. R., Shariat, M., et al. (2008). Effects of a psychological intervention on depression in infertile couples. *International Journal of Gynecology & Obstetrics*, 101(3):248–52.

[17] Johansson, M. Adolfsson, A., Berg, M., Francis, J., Hogström, L., Olof P., et al. (2009). Quality of life for couples 4–5.5 years after unsuccessful IVF treatment. *Acta Obstetricia et Gynecologica Scandinavica*, 88(3):291–300.

[18] Meyers, M., Weinshel, M., Scharf, C., Kezur, D., Diamond, R., Rait, D. S. (1995). An Infertility Primer for Family Therapists: II. Working with Couples Who Struggle with Infertility. *Family Process,* 34(2): 231–40.

[19] Mohiyiddeen, L., Cerra, C. (2017). Biopsychosocial Aspects of Infertility. In: Edozien LC, O'Brien PMS, editors. Biopsychosocial Factors in Obstetrics and Gynaecology. 1st ed. Cambridge University Press: 110–20. Available from: https://www.cambridge.org/core/product/identifier/9781316341261% 23CN-bp-14/type/book_part.

In: Obstetric and Gynecology Case Report ISBN: 978-1-53616-711-5
Editor: Dwiana Ocviyanti

Chapter 14

INFERTILITY DUE TO POLYCYSTIC OVARY SYNDROME

Sri Suryo Adiyanti* and Suzanna Immanuel
Department of Clinical Pathology, Faculty of Medicine, Universitas Indonesia, Jakarta, Indonesia

ABSTRACT

Polycystic ovary syndrome (PCOS) is commonly observed in women of reproductive age. This syndrome presents with symptoms such as amenorrhea, hirsutism, and obesity. Impairment of feedback between the hypothalamus–pituitary axis and ovary increases the secretion of estrogen, decreasing the secretion of follicle-stimulating hormone (FSH). Herein, we report the case of a 29-year-old married women who sought fertility consultation at our intuition. The following laboratory results were obtained: an elevated luteinizing hormone (LH) level during the follicular stage (22.390 mIU/mL) and an FSH/LH ratio of 4.6 (elevated >2.5). Such findings are indicative of PCOS. Moreover, the patient presented with amenorrhea and irregular menstruation. Her last menstrual period was 1.5 years back. The patient has been experiencing primary infertility for 3

* Correspounding Author's Email: theayukari@yahoo.com.

years. Ultrasonography revealed the following results: retroflexion on the cavum uteri, uterus of normal size, endometrial thickness of 11 mm, and polycystic ovaries.

Keywords: polycystic ovary syndrome, infertility, obesity, estrogen, insulin resistance

INTRODUCTION

Polycystic ovary syndrome (PCOS) is an endocrine disorder observed in 5%–10% of young women of reproductive ageand is characterized by variations and complexity of metabolic and endocrine disorders [1, 2]. In 1935, PCOS was initially described by Stein and Leventhal as a triad of amenorrhea, hirsutism, and obesity among women with multiple cysts in the ovary [3, 4]. During the reproductive age, PCOS is associated with infertility, abnormal bleeding, miscarriage, and gestational complications; therefore, it significantly interferes with the quality of life of women during their reproductive age and contributes to morbidity and mortality during the menopause period. The clinical signs of PCOS persist until the menopause period, which causes delayed menopause. PCOS patients have high prevalence of hysterectomy as well as diabetes and hypertension [5]. To date, the cause of PCOS is unknown, and such condition may be an autosomal dominant inheritance [4]. The pathogenesis of PCOS is not yet fully elucidated. However, insulin resistance, hyperandrogenemia, anovulation, and polycystic ovary are associated with its pathophysiology [6].

The clinical signs of PCOS constitute changes in lipid profile and lipoprotein levels, which include slight elevation in cholesterol and triglyceride levels and decrease in LDL, HDL, and apolipoprotein A-1 levels. These changes may be influenced by body weight, diet, and ethnicity [4]. Hyperandrogenemia plays a major role; however, hyperinsulinemia (insulin resistance) is a more significant factor [4, 5]. Insulin resistance induces changes in lipolysis response, which is impairment of the suppression of fatty acid release from adipose tissues; thus, the free fatty acid level increases. As a result, liver triglyceride synthesis also increases [4, 5, 7]. Approximately 40%–50% women with PCOS present with android/central obesity and high waist-to-hip ratio. Obesity could worsen insulin resistance and increase the risk of developing diabetes and cardiovascular diseases [4, 5]. In women with hyperandrogenemia and chronic anovulation, the diagnosis of PCOS should be considered after other endocrine disorders are ruled out. Hyperandrogenemia and chronic anovulation are the most common clinical signs of PCOS [3].

PCOS is a syndrome that cannot be diagnosed by conducting only a single diagnostic test. Diagnostic criteria for such conditions have been developed and used worldwide. However, the diagnosis could be challenging because there are variations in the symptoms based on age and changes with time. The clinical signs commonly include amenorrhea, which resolves within years, and progressive worsening of hirsutism [3, 7, 8].

The Rotterdam consensus on the diagnosis of PCOS should include two of three criteria listed below [3, 8]:

1) Oligo or chronic anovulation manifesting as oligomenorrhea or amenorrhea
2) Clinical or biochemical signs showing hyperandrogenism (hirsutism, acne, baldness, and elevated free fatty acid or total testosterone levels)
3) Polycystic ovary based on ultrasonography ($\geq$12 follicles with a diameter of 2–9 mm) and/or elevation of ovary volume >10 mL)

Other etiologies include congenital adrenal hyperplasia, androgen-secreting tumors, and Cushing syndrome.

The following information should be considered: reproductive history (menarche, previous and current cycle, oligo/amenorrhea, miscarriage and infertility), presentation of androgenic signs (acne, hirsutism, and alopecia), weight changes, and lifestyle habits (eating and sports habits and smoking and alcohol history). Family history of PCOS and diabetes, obesity, hirsutism, and early baldness, which is prominent in men, must also be assessed. Physical examination of women suspected with PCOS include weight examination (body mass index and hip-to-waist ratio), assessment of the presence of acne and hirsutism, and blood pressure measurement [3, 8-10].

Laboratory examination reveals elevated androgen levels, and abnormalities in menstrual cycle or polycystic ovaries are identified on ultrasonography. These findings met the diagnostic criteria. Although luteinizing hormone (LH)/follicle-stimulating hormone (FSH) examination is not important, some clinicians still recommend such tests. After diagnosis, fasting glucose and lipid examinations are recommended. Other tests (prolactin, testosterone, DHEA-S, and corticotropin-stimulated 17 alpha-hydroxyprogesterone) might be required based on clinical signs to rule out differential diagnosis [3]. Insulin resistance could occur; therefore, fasting glucose and insulin levels should be measured to evaluate for hyperinsulinemia. Insulin resistance could be measured using the homeostasis model assessment-insulin resistance (HOMA-IR) and by measuring the level of accumulated insulin and calculating fasting glucose/fasting insulin ratio [6, 10].

$$\text{HOMA-IR} = \text{fasting insulin (mU/L)} \times \text{fasting glucose (mmol/L)}$$

The study of Lee has shown that a HOMA-IR score of >3.29 and Wahrenberg score of >3.99 are indicative of insulin resistance [8]. Muharam has revealed that insulin resistance is diagnosed when fasting glucose/fasting insulin level is <10.1 [11].

CASE ILLUSTRATION

A 29-year-old married woman visited our clinic for infertility consultation. Laboratory findings revealed the following: anti-Mullerian hormone level, 8.37 ng/mL; elevated LH level, 22.390 mIU/mL; FSH level, 4.8 mIU/mL; prolactin level, 14.56 ng/mL; and estradiol level, 35.22 pg/mL. The patient was previously diagnosed with PCOS. Her LH/FSH ratio was

4.6 (elevated >2.5), which further supported the diagnosis of PCOS. . Moreover, the following results were obtained: fasting glucose level, 88 mg/dL; 2-h postprandial glucose level, 86 mg/dL; fasting insulin level, 9 μIU/mL; and 2-h postprandial insulin level, 40.4 μIU/mL.

The examination of LH, FSG, and estradiol levels is conducted during the follicular phase. The patient presented with menstrual abnormalities, she experienced amenorrhea, and was previously assessed by a gynecologist. She was then diagnosed with PCOS. Her last menstrual period was 1.5 years back, and the patient had been experiencing primary infertility for 3 years. Ultrasonography revealed retroflexion of the cavum uteri, uterus of normal size, endometrial thickness of 11 mm, and polycystic ovaries.

DISCUSSION

Fasting glucose, 2-h postprandial glucose, fasting insulin, and 2-h postprandial insulin levels were examined to assess insulin resistance. The patient was then found to have an HOMA-IR score of 8.8 (≥4.39), indicating that the patient had insulin resistance, which is typically observed in PCOS as result of a defect in insulin receptor signaling. According to Muharam, a fasting glucose/fasting insulin level of 9.7 (<10.1) indicates insulin resistance and supports the diagnosis of PCOS [11].

Moreover, changes in LH and FSH levels are noted. In patients with PCOS, pulsatile secretion of LH is observed, whereas no changes are noted in FSH levels. Therefore, the LH/FSH ratio could increase greater than 2.5, even if the ovarian cycle is normal. This value was within normal limits which is the ratio of LH/FSH not exceed more than 2.5 in approximately 10%–20% of the patients. The feedback process between the core (hypothalamus–hypophysis) and ovary is impaired; thus, the estrogen level will remain high, and there will be inadequate production of FSH [12].

According to the Rotterdam international consensus in 2003, the patient was diagnosed with PCOS as two of three criteria were met: chronic anovulation (which usually manifests as oligomenorrhea or amenorrhea) and polycystic ovary (which is observed on ultrasonography and is characterized by ≥12 follicles with a size of 2–9 mm on in each ovary and/or increase in ovarium volume >10 mL). Women with PCOS do not have single egg cells, and there are numerous cells (15–30) that grow together in the ovary. These cells do not mature and gradually develop into cysts.

PCOS can be easily diagnosed on imaging such as USG. That is, an egg cell that is >9 mL with more than 8 mL of peripheral cystic structure (<10 mm) on a sonographic plane and is surrounded by stromal mass elevation (>25% ovarium volume) is observed [4]. Normally, few egg cells are produced every month; however, not all cells reach maturity. In fact, only one reaches maturity and is then released. When this cell increases in size, other cells shrink. This single egg cell is referred to as egg cell or dominant follicle. A healthy ovary comprises one dominant follicle and other (<10) small follicles. In patients with PCOS, there are no dominant follicles; however, there are numerous egg cells (15–30 growing egg cells in the ovary), which can further develop into cysts [13] (Figure 1).

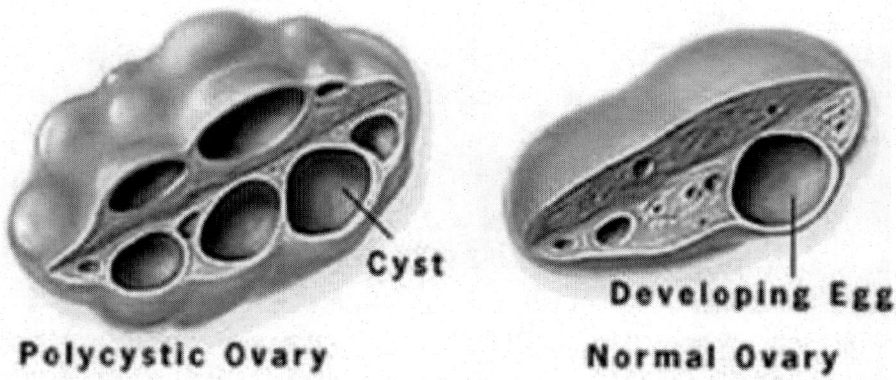

Figure 1. Comparison between a polycystic ovary (left) and a normal ovary (right) [13].

The patient's FSH/LH ratio was 4.6 (elevated >2.5), which was elevated. Such a finding is a result of the lack of a dominant follicle formed during the follicular phase, which is replaced by multiple small follicles that are not capable of ovulation. This patient did not menstruate for 1.5 years, therefore, the examination is considered done on follicular phase. The egg cell does not maturate and is not released to the tube and then to the uterus. The ovary will continue producing estrogen and testosterone; however, there will be over secretion of progesterone when ovulation ceases. Most women with PCOS have an irregular menstrual cycle [13].

Patients with suspected PCOS are usually advised to undergo testosterone, lipid profile (total cholesterol, HDL, LDL, and TG), and blood glucose examinations. The first-line therapy for PCOS is lifestyle modification, which is effective in managing PCOS as it reduces obesity and insulin resistance. Moreover, it can help treat endocrine problems and irregular menstrual cycles. Pharmacological treatment includes the use of anti-androgen drugs, oral contraceptives, or progesterone medications to enhance normal menstrual cycle and produce insulin-sensitizing agents, such as metformin, to lower insulin levels [3, 5, 9, 12].

CONCLUSION

Here in, we report the case of a woman of reproductive age who presented with primary infertility attributed to PCOS. The patient was diagnosed based on the following findings: chronic anovulation, polycystic ovary based on ultrasonography, LH/FSH ratio of 4.6, and HOMA-IR score of 8.8. Women with PCOS can be accompanied by android/central obesity and high waist-to-hip ratio. Obesity could worsen insulin resistance and increase the risk of developing diabetes and cardiovascular diseases. In women with hyperandrogenemia and chronic anovulation, the diagnosis of PCOS should be considered after other endocrine disorders are ruled out. Hyperandrogenemia and chronic anovulation are the most common clinical signs of PCOS. Patient needs to be monitored routinely check for the lipid profile and glucose tests based on insulin resistance as tha main factor that plays main role in PCOS.

References

[1] Hart, R. Hickey M. Franks S. (2004). Definitions, prevalence and symptoms of polycystic ovaries and polycystic ovary syndrome. *Best Pract Res Clin Obstet Gynaecol,* 18(5):671-683.

[2] Azziz, R. Woods K. S., Rayna R. et al. (2004). The Prevalence and Features of the Polycystic Ovary Syndrome in an Unselected Population. *J Clin Endocrinol Metab*, 89(6):2745-2749.

[3] Farquhar, C. & Johnson, N. (2008). Understanding polycystic ovary syndrome. *Best Practice Journal (BPJ), 2*: 7-13.

[4] Lobo, R. A. & Carmina, E. (2000).The importance of diagnosing the polycystic ovary syndrome. *Annals of Internal Medicine*, *132*: 989-993.

[5] Carmina, E. & Lobo, R. A. (1999). Polycystic ovary syndrome (PCOS): arguably the most common endocrinopathy is associated with significant morbidity in women. *The Journal of Endocrinology and Metabolism*, *84*: 1897-1899.

[6] Immanuel, S. (2010). Patogenesis dan Diagnosis Laboratorik Sindrom Ovarium Polikistik. In: Oesman F, editors (Eds.). *Pendidikan Berkesinambungan Patologi Klinik*. (edition, pp.140-161). Jakarta: Balai Penerbit FKUI.

[7] Marx, T. L. & Mehta, A. E. (2003). Polycystic ovary syndrome: pathogenesis and treatment over the short and long term. *Cleveland Clinic Journal of Medicine*, *70*: 31-45.

[8] Lee, J. M., Okumura, M. J., Davis, M. M., Herman, W. H., & Gurney, J. G. (2006). Prevalence and determinants of insulin resistance among US adolescents: a population-based study. *Diabetes Care*, *29*: 2427-2432.

[9] Muharam, R., Kdarusman, Y. & Jacoeb, T. Z. (2001). Sudarsono S. Mengetahui Nisbah Gula Darah Puasa/Insulin Puasapada Ovarium Polikistik. *Maj Obstet Ginekol Indones*, *25*: 109-119.

[10] Maharani, L. & Wratsangka, L. (2002). Sindrom Ovarium Polikistik: Permasalahandan Penatalaksanaannya. *Journal Kedokteran Trisakti*, *21*: 98-103.

[11] Women's Health Program, Monash University. (2010). *Polycyctic Ovarian Syndrome (PCOS).* [Internet]. Available at http://womens health.med.monash.edu.au. Downloaded on April 19th, 2013.

[12] Ehrmann, D. A. (2005). Polycystic ovary syndrome. *New England Journal of Medicine*, *352*: 1223-1236.

[13] Boyle, J. & Teede, H. J. (2012). Polycystic ovary syndrome: an update. *Australian family physician*. *10*: 752-756.

In: Obstetric and Gynecology Case Report
Editor: Dwiana Ocviyanti
ISBN: 978-1-53616-711-5

Chapter 15

AGGRESSIVE MANAGEMENT OF LOW-RISK ENDOMETRIAL CANCER IN INFERTILE PATIENTS OF LOW SOCIOECONOMIC STATUS

Yuli Achmad Saputra[1,*] *and Dwiana Ocviyanti*[2]
[1]Faculty of Medicine, Universitas Indonesia, Jakarta, Indonesia
[2]Department of Obstetric and Gynecology, Faculty of Medicine, Universitas Indonesia, Dr. Cipto Mangunkusumo Hospital, Jakarta, Indonesia

ABSTRACT

Aggressive management of endometrial cancer often involves hysterectomy, a procedure where a part of the uterus is taken out to eliminate the cancer. This procedure results in secondary infertility and this may cause significant morbidity, especially in patients who wishes to have children. A 29-year-old woman presented with a chief complaint of vaginal bleeding.

* Corresponding Author's Email: saputrh@gmail.com.

Curettage and hysteroscopy revealed a low-risk endometrial cancer. The patient was first given conservative therapy to preserve the uterus. After 1 year of treatment, her condition did not improve. The patient was of low socioeconomic status and was unable to afford in vitro fertilization. She decided to undergo hysterectomy, even though she was of childbearing age. Secondary infertility due to medical procedures significantly impacts the patient's biology, psychology, and social factors. This patient's decision to undergo aggressive treatment for endometrial cancer is influenced by her disadvantaged background. A patient's socioeconomic status influences her decision making and affects her quality of life. This case illustrates how a patient's socioeconomic status influences clinical decision making and progression of the disease. The clinician must appreciate socioeconomic factors that may influence a patient's preference in managing endometrial cancer.

Keywords: endometrial cancer, socioeconomic influence, clinical decision making

INTRODUCTION

Uterine cancer is one of the most common gynecologic malignancies in developed countries. The prevalence of this uterine cancer is steadily increasing. This cancer often occurs in young women, causing significant biopsychosocial morbidity. The most common presenting sign is abnormal uterine bleeding. However, a substantial number of cases present without any signs or symptoms [1].

Patients are usually diagnosed in the early stage, when the tumor is still confined to the uterus. The treatment for endometrial carcinoma is hysterectomy and removal of both fallopian tubes and ovaries (bilateral salpingo-oophorectomy), and other adjuvant treatment according to the stage of the cancer. This treatment regimen is effective in most cases. The five-year survival rate is good, ranging from 74%-91% if diagnosed in the early stage. In women who want to preserve their fertility, hormonal therapy has been used in early stage of the disease, and can be effective [1].

Murray et al. discuss patients' preferences and factors that influence patients' decision making [2, 3]. This case report discusses hysterectomy and salpingo-oophorectomy performed in patients in child bearing age with low socioeconomic status. This case report suggests that the main factors that influence patient decision making are perceived quality of life and socioeconomic factors. The report focuses on how socioeconomic factors may influence patient's care. The limitation of this report is that it is based on a case found in Indonesia, a developed country, the conditions might be different in other countries.

CASE REPORT

A 29-year-old woman was referred to from Carolus Hospital with endometrial cancer. The patient had a history of vaginal bleeding for 2.5 months. To confirm the diagnosis, pathology specimens were collected from the patient, and she was diagnosed with endometrial carcinoma with good differentiation (grade 1). She was treated with high-dose progestin (600 mg/day) and was evaluated every 3 months.

The patient had been admitted to dr. Cipto Mangunkusumo (RSCM) Hospital 1 year before admission to our hospital because of absence of menstruation for the previous 2 months. She was diagnosed with oligomenorrhea with obesity, insulin resistance, and primary infertility and was treated with Drospirenone 3 mg and Ethyinl estradiol 0.02 mg (Yaz) one tablet a day for menstrual regulation and metformin 500 mg thrice a day.

At follow-up 3 months later, resection hysteroscopy showed atypical hyperplasia and squamous metaplasia. Magnetic resonance imaging revealed diffuse restricted endometrial thickening with infiltration into the myometrium in the left posterior fundus uteri. Repeat hysteroscopy revealed an endometrium highly influenced by progesterone and no malignancy. The patient was diagnosed with endometrium cancer 1A.

Immunohistochemical analysis was performed to test for the mismatch repair (MMR) genes MSH2, MLH1, MSH6, and PMS2. A positive result was found for the secondary protein MSH6, which indicates a mutation in the MMR gene. Ultrasonography revealed a 14 × 9 cm echogenic mass with irregular edges that was mostly formed by the endometrial malignancy.

Because repeat hysteroscopy showed no significant improvement in the patient's condition, a laparoscopic total hysterectomy accompanied by left salpingo-oophorectomy was performed. The procedure went uneventfully.

DISCUSSION

Aggressive Management of Endometrial Cancer

Most patients with endometrial carcinoma undergo hysterectomy. The surgical staging includes median incisions, peritoneal rinses, exploration of metastases, total hysterectomy, bilateral salpingo-oophorectomy, pelvic lymph node lymphadenectomy, and para-aortic lymphadenectomy. Patients with endometrial cancer must be surgically staged according to the joint 2010 International Federation of Gynecology and Obstetrics/Tumor Lymph Node and Metastases (TNM) Classification system. In the 2010 classification system, the definition of stage 1 was changed to include only two substages: 1A (tumor limited to the endometrium or invades less than one-half of the myometrium) and 1B (tumor invades one-half or more of the myometrium). In the previous surgical staging system for endometrial carcinoma, stage 1 had three substages: 1A (tumor limited to the endometrium), 1B (tumor invades less than one-half of the myometrium), and 1C (tumor invades one-half or more of the myometrium). It appears that the 2010 staging system is able to predict prognosis better than the previous system [4]. Lymph node evaluation should also be performed, as the involvement of the lymph nodes is one of the most important prognostic factors for endometrial carcinoma. Sentinel lymph node biopsy is commonly performed. The role of this procedure, however, is still limited. A study of more than 28,000 women who underwent surgical staging for endometrial cancer between 2011 and 2015 reported that 32.9% had no nodal assessment, 62.3% had lymphadenectomy, and 4.8% had sentinel lymph node biopsy. Successful mapping of at least one sentinel lymph node was achieved in 86% of patients, and the sensitivity of sentinel lymph node biopsy was 97.2% [4].

Vaginal hysterectomy is not generally recommended for endometrial carcinoma because it precludes examination of the abdomen and lymph nodes for metastases. A surgical approach may be appropriate for women who are poor candidates for major abdominal surgery. In this population, retrospective series have reported that vaginal hysterectomy is associated with a low rate of perioperative complications and a 5 to 10-year disease-specific survival rate of 80% or higher. However, because staging is uncertain in these women, it is not possible to compare these data with survival rates for other women [5]. In women who undergo vaginal hysterectomy, BSO should also be performed. Women who are at intermediate (grade 3 tumors or above) or greater risk of disease recurrence may be advised to have adjuvant radiation therapy.

Secondary Infertility Due to Procedure

It is known that hysterectomy is associated with infertility [6].A common complication of this procedure is depression secondary to loss of fertility. Leppert et al. [6] analyzed the effects of hysterectomy on the patient, including depression. The study sample was 1140 women undergoing hysterectomy for benign indications who were interviewed before and after surgery up to 2 years of follow-up. The outcomes were psychological distress, anxiety, depression, anger, and confusion. The outcomes were measured 12 and 24 months postoperatively. Of the sample, 10.5% answered "yes" to questions such as "Before you were told you needed a hysterectomy, would you have wanted a (or another) child?" Women who desired a child or another child were usually nulliparous; waited longer before having surgery; were more likely to have endometriosis; and had higher levels of depression, anger, confusion, and anxiety. The women also were more than twice as likely to have seen a mental health professional for anxiety or depression in the 3 months before surgery. These conditions persisted throughout the 2-year follow-up period. The patient in this case report fulfilled the criteria for high-risk hysterectomy: young, nulliparous, and had high levels of anxiety and depression. The issue of loss of fertility should be discussed candidly with women considering hysterectomy and those who express ambivalence or sadness. Those facing the loss of childbearing ability may benefit from exploration of fertility-sparing treatments.

Factors Influencing Medical Decision Making: The Role of Socioeconomic Factors

Medical decision making is influenced by several factors. The most important factors affecting patient care are the patient's race and socioeconomic status [7]. A study by van Ryn and Burke [7] analyzed the effect of the patient's race and socioeconomic status on the physician's perception of and attitude toward the patient, controlling for age, sex, race, frailty or sickness, depression, knowledge, social assertiveness, and physician characteristics. Ryn and Burke states that the physician's perception of the patient was influenced by the patient's sociodemographic characteristics [8]. Physicians tended to perceive members of minority ethnic groups and low and middle socioeconomic groups more negatively in a number of dimensions compared with Caucasian patients and patients with upper-socioeconomic status. The patient's race was associated with the physician's assessment of the patient's intelligence, feeling of affiliation toward the patient, and beliefs about the patient's risky behavior and adherence to medical advice. The patient's socioeconomic status was associated with the physician's perceptions of his or her personality, abilities, behavioral tendencies, and role.

In our case, the patient is a housewife and her husband worked as a fisherman with total income of less than 2 million Indonesia Rupiah per month. The patient is classified as having low socioeconomic status, according to Indonesian Central Agency on Statistic. This may influence the physician's decision to perform hysterectomy if the physician perceives that the patient cannot afford *in vitro* fertilization. Physicians should recognize this bias and treat patients according to their objective condition.

The patient's education also plays an important role in his or her treatment and the issue of informed consent. Studies have shown that patients with less education tend to have less understanding of their medical condition and tend to follow patriarchal decision making rather than shared decision making with the primary care provider. The patient may follow the physician's advice regardless of his or her personal attitude toward the subject. To solve this problem, Sudore et al. developed a method for vulnerable patients called modified informed consent [9]. With this method, the physician gives informed consent to the patient and assesses the patient's comprehension before determining if the patient is giving consent or not. The consent form contains comprehension statement, patients have to respond with "true," "false," or "I don't know" and patients have to respond correctly to all statements before giving consent, if patients responded incorrectly to any statement, that statement will be repeated until comprehension is achieved.

This research found that patients who have not completed primary education and those of lower socioeconomic status have poorer comprehension of the procedure that they are going to undergo. Modified informed consent must be provided in order for the patient to have adequate knowledge and understanding regarding the problem. The research addressed several problems regarding the informed consent process, including improving the readability and design of the consent forms and providing ample time for discussion of information required for consent. Understanding is improved by using an iterative educational strategy in which formal assessment of understanding is linked with repeated passes through targeted education until the patient has adequate understanding. The consent form must also contain a question aimed at the care provider, to make sure the care provider knows the level of understanding and knowledge of the patient regarding the procedure.

In this case, because the patient had low socioeconomic status and low education, she may have had low knowledge regarding the possible consequences of the procedure for childbearing. Lack of clear information may lead a patient to patriarchal decision making that may cause psychosocial morbidity in the patient.

Fertility Problem Stress

Studies have shown that infertility may affect biopsychosocial aspects of patients. Schmid et al. showed the effects of infertility on patients [10]. These effects include marital stress, social stress, and personal stress. Multivariate analysis revealed that women reported more fertility problem stress than men. The univariate F-test revealed that women reported significantly more personal and social stress than men. However, there was no difference between men and women in the impact of infertility on marital stress. Findings from the study of Schmid et al. showed that fertility problem stress was primarily associated with the patient's rating of the importance of patient-centered care. Personal and marital stress was associated with higher importance ratings for patient-centered care in both men and women. Higher marital stress for men predicted a higher importance rating for discussions about adoption with the medical staff. Marital benefits were also associated with higher importance ratings for patient-centered care. Increasing age decreases the psychosocial stress associated with infertility [11].

CONCLUSION

Loss of childbearing potential is one of the consequences of hysterectomy. Adequate informed consent and education regarding the possible consequences of this procedure are needed. In addition, psychosocial support for patients is needed to boost their psychological and social conditions. Physicians should recognize potential bias due to the patient's psychosocial factors that might influence their clinical judgment.

REFERENCES

[1] Morice, P., Leary, A., Creutzberg, C., Abu-Rustum, N., Darai, E. Endometrial cancer. (2016). *The Lancet*, 387:1094-1108.

[2] Murray, E., Pollack, L., White, M., Lo B. (2007). Clinical decision-making: Patients' preferences and experiences. *Patient Education and Counseling*, 65:189-196.

[3] Adolescent Pregnancy Guidelines. (2015). *SOGC Clinical Practice Guideline*:327.

[4] Daraï, E., Dubernard, G., Bats, A. S., Heitz, D., Mathevet, P., Marret, H., et al. (2015). Sentinel node biopsy for the management of early stage endometrial cancer: Long-term results of the SENTI-ENDO study. *Gynecologic Oncology*, 136: 54-59.

[5] Wright, J. D., Burke, W. M., Tergas, A.I., Hou, J. Y., Huang, Y., Hu JC, et al. (2016). Comparative effectiveness of minimally invasive hysterectomy for endometrial cancer. *Journal of Clinical Oncology: Official Journal of the American Society of Clinical Oncology*, 34:1087-1096.

[6] Leppert, P. C., Legro, R. S., Kjerulff, K. H. (2007). Hysterectomy and loss of fertility: Implications for women's mental health. *Journal of Psychosomatic Research*, 63:269-274.

[7] van Ryn, M., Burke, J. (2000). The effect of patient race and socio-economic status on physicians' perceptions of patients. *Social Science & Medicine*, 50: 813-828.

[8] Bowe, C. M., Armstrong, E. (2017). Assessment for systems learning: a holistic assessment framework to support decision making across the medical education continuum. *Academic Medicine*, 92: 585-592.

[9] Sudore, R. L., Landefeld, C. S., Williams, B. A., Barnes, D. E., Lindquist, K., Schillinger, D. (2006). Use of a modified informed consent process among vulnerable patients: a descriptive study. *Journal of General Internal Medicine*, 21:867-873.

[10] Upchurch, D. M., Stein, J., Greendale, G. A., Chyu, L., Tseng, C. H., Huang, M. H., et al. (2015). A longitudinal investigation of race, socioeconomic status, and psychosocial mediators of allostatic load in midlife women: findings from the study of women's health across the nation. *Psychosomatic Medicine*, 77: 402-412.

[11] Luk, B. H. K., Loke, A. Y. (2015). The impact of infertility on the psychological well-being, marital relationships, sexual relationships, and quality of life of couples: a systematic review. *Journal of Sex & Marital Therapy*, 41: 610-625.

In: Obstetric and Gynecology Case Report ISBN: 978-1-53616-711-5
Editor: Dwiana Ocviyanti

Chapter 16

BIOPSYCHOSOCIAL APPROACH IN A WOMAN WITH CHRONIC PELVIC PAIN, ABNORMAL UTERINE BLEEDING, AND PRIMARY SUBFERTILITY DUE TO ENDOMETRIOSIS

Aginta Ginting** and Dwiana Ocviyanti

Department of Obstetric and Gynecology, Faculty of Medicine, Universitas Indonesia, Dr. Cipto Mangunkusumo Hospital, Jakarta, Indonesia

ABSTRACT

The presence of normal endometrial mucosa outside of the uterine cavity is known as endometriosis. Endometriosis patients complain of several symptoms, including chronic pelvic pain in 50% of patients, subfertility in 30% – 50%, and dysmenorrhea in 12% – 32% [1, 2]. Chronic

* Corresponding Author's E-mail: gintingaginta@gmail.com.

pain and subfertility can affect the psychological status of endometriosis patients. Adequate counseling can improve the patients' and their spouses' acceptance of the condition and improve treatment compliance. A 31-year-old woman presented with chief complaints of dysmenorrhea with a Visual Analog Scale (VAS) score of 6, anemia due to abnormal uterine bleeding, and primary infertility for 6 years. The patient had suffered from pelvic pain for 10 years. She used to work but resigned because of her condition. She also admitted that the symptoms affect her daily activity and social life. The subfertility causes her to avoid meeting friends and family. The physical examination and ultrasound identified adenomyosis and a right endometriosis cyst. The patient was hospitalized for transfusion and given an analgetic and dienogest. Dysmenorrhea had affected the patient's daily activities for approximately 10 years and had worsened in the past 2 years. She received medical treatment, and the pain decreased. However, she had not been regularly taking her medication recently, and she returned to the hospital because of abnormal uterine bleeding and pain. The management for endometriosis is to relieve the symptoms and increase the chance for fertility. Psychologically, the pain and the frequent admissions to the hospital affected her life, causing depression and eliminating her social life. Adequate counseling provided to the patient and her husband regarding her condition and understanding the possibility of treatment for pain and infertility may decrease the psychological problem.

Keywords: biopsychosocial, endometriosis, chronic pelvic pain, subfertility

INTRODUCTION

As previously mentioned, the presence of normal endometrial mucosa outside of the uterine cavity is known as endometriosis [1, 2]. It is usually diagnosed in women over 30 years old, which is the reproductive age and affects 5% – 10% women in their thirties [2]. Endometriosis patients complain of several symptoms, including chronic pelvic pain in 50% of patients, subfertility in 30% – 50%, and dysmenorrhea in 12% – 32% [1, 2]. In RSCM, 82.5% of cases reported chronic pelvic pain, 81% of cases reported dysmenorrhea, and 33.7% of cases reported subfertility [3].

The benign invasion of the endometrium into the myometrium, which produces a diffusely enlarged uterus that microscopically exhibits ectopic nonneoplastic endometrial glands and stroma surrounded by a hypertrophic and hyperplastic myometrium is known as adenomyosis [4, 5]. Adenomyosis usually causes subfertility [5].

Furthermore, adenomyosis can be diagnosed through pathology examination by hysterectomy specimen. Hence, subfertile patient examination cannot be evaluated. Moreover, the patient with subfertility condition rarely gets pregnant. Until today, no data were found to evaluate the relationship between adenomyosis and subfertile conditions [5].

The aim of management is to alleviate the pain and increase the possibility for fertility. The medical treatment is not to resorb the lesion because the lesion can recur after the treatment is stopped. The treatment should be individually specific based on the chief complaint and the expected result. A systematic literature review has shown that if amenorrhea occurs, the tolerability, side effects, and cost widely vary, and there are no statistical differences between the various available drugs to relieve the pain [6]. Medical treatments for endometriosis aim to reduce the production of endogenous estrogen or induce the differentiation of endometrium using progestin. Clinical evidence points to the clear and deleterious effect of uninterrupted ovulatory cycles on the development and persistence of endometriosis.

The main goal of the treatment is to inhibit the ovulation and to achieve a stable steroid hormone concentration [6]. Some evidence of an association can also be derived from reports of infertile women achieving pregnancy after being treated for endometriosis. The first agents utilized for this purpose were GnRH-A.

Both medical and surgical treatments offer opportunities for disease stabilization and regression. The initial therapy for focal endometriosis involves hormonal suppression with Combination Oral Contraception (COC), particularly for female adolescents in whom preserving fertility is important. Adolescents may represent a subset of patients with endometriosis whose lesions are completely treatable with hormonal therapy [7].

There are many considerations in the treatment of endometriosis. For example, GnRH agonists are drugs with higher costs and more troublesome side effects. Although they are very effective against endometriosis-related pain and also contribute to the occurrence of many successful pregnancies and deliveries, their use is associated with frequent and intolerable hypoestrogenic side effects, including vasomotor syndrome, genital atrophy, and mood instability. These drugs should only be used for a short period of time among adolescents whose symptoms do not improve with the continuous use of COC. GnRH agonists also have a negative impact on bone health and a possible negative influence on cardiovascular health [6].

All components of chronic pain, which is a biopsychosocial condition, should be evidence-based. It requires multi modal and interdisciplinary treatment [7, 8]. The "biopsychosocial model" of care is defined in Relieving Pain's glossary to evaluate multiple aspects such as the biological, psychological, and social dimensions of illness and disease. The biopsychosocial model aims to provide the basis of the disease so we can understand the basis and can threat the main problem. It provided the patient with her social context. The model states that health and disease are the result of interactions among biological, psychological, and social factors [7].

The biopsychosocial approach shows that the concept of pain cannot divide physical or psychosocial elements. [7] Integrated pain management defined it functionally as follows [7]:

1. Informed by evidence
2. Patient-centered and reaffirms the importance of the healing, covenantal partnership between practitioner and patient
3. Focused on the whole person-mind, body, and spirit in the context of the individual's community/environment
4. Inclusive of all appropriate therapeutic approaches and healthcare professionals to reduce pain, improve function, achieve optimal health and healing, and provide physical emotional rehabilitation
5. Individualized, recognizing that no single treatment or paradigm may be perfectly suited for every patient, particularly those in chronic pain.

Biopsychosocial approach can find the symptoms of endometriosis and subfertility. Statistics in United States indicate that 15% of all couples who are subfertile will experience the frustration of infertility in their relationship [8]. The high incidence of subfertility almost guarantees that the complex emotional roller coaster related to subfertility faced by individuals and couples will be an issue in some facet of their counseling.

The effort required to cope with subfertility may be demanding and stressful: finding the time to complete all of the medical examinations, deciding how much money to invest in the treatments, and determining how long to battle insurance companies for reimbursement for the related medical procedures [9]. There can be a tremendous sense of frustration and anger toward professionals in the medical field for failing to fix the uncertainty.

Several couples felt that their subfertile condition had been misunderstood by their friends and family. About 80% of infertile couples reported receiving negative comments from their environment. Because of the uncomfortable condition, they may distance themselves from their social lives [10].

CASE ILLUSTRATION

A 31-year-old female presented with the chief complaints of pelvic pain with a VAS score of 6, anemia due to abnormal uterine bleeding, and primary infertility for 6 years. The patient admitted that she had bleeding from the vagina for the 2 weeks prior to admission. This was her second experience of receiving transfusion due to bleeding in the last 4 months. The patient had complained of dysmenorrhea for the past 10 years, which had worsened in the 2 years prior to admission. She had received medical therapy 6 months earlier. She did not display dyspareunia, defecation, or dysuria. The patient had previously visited several doctors for these issues until she was referred to our hospital. The patient had been taking dienogest for the past 6 months, and she admitted that it relieved her pain. However, she had not been taking the drug regularly for the past 3 months. The patient had never had an operation before. She had not previously been pregnant and not yet been evaluated for her subfertility condition. Despite her subfertility, the patient was concerned about the pain; however, she still wished to become pregnant in the future.

The patient is a housewife. She used to work but resigned because of her condition. She originally complained about pain during her period and being unable to perform her daily activities and having to take medication during her period. More recently, she also complained about weakness and prolonged vaginal bleeding.

A physical examination revealed that her general status was within normal limits but her conjunctiva was pale. On palpation, there was a solid and immobile mass in the abdomen one finger below the navel. Gynecological examination found that fluxus was positive, that there were no nodules, and that the uterine was globular and immobile. The ultrasound examination revealed a hyperechoic appearance with an unclear border size of 62 × 73mm at the posterior corpus, which corresponded to adenomyosis. There was a cystic mass on the right adnexa with a ground glass appearance size of 46 × 52mm, which corresponded with an endometriosis cyst. The laboratory results reported a hemoglobin level of 6.9gr/dl. The patient was hospitalized to receive a transfusion and was given an analgetic and dienogest.

DISCUSSION

Endometriosis can display symptoms of chronic pelvic pain and subfertility. In 2004, the American College of Obstetrics and Gynecology defined chronic pelvic pain as cyclical pelvic pain lasting at least 6 months that affects daily activity and requires medical intervention [11]. Chronic pelvic pain affects quality of life. However, patients usually try to treat themselves with over-the-counter drugs.

Infertility is the other symptom of patients with endometriosis. Infertility causes the patients to feel incomplete as women and can cause depression, further removing these women from their social lives [10].

The goal of therapy in patients with endometriosis is to relieve the symptoms, not to eliminate the lesions. Therefore, the first line of therapy is pain control. If the endometriosis is causing infertility, surgery is an option, even if recurrence is possible.

In this patient, dysmenorrhea had affected her daily activities for approximately 10 years and had worsened over the last 2 years. She had been taking over-the-counter drugs for several years. She had been diagnosed with endometriosis 1 year earlier. She received medical treatment and her pain decreased. However, recently, she had not been regularly taking her medication, and she returned to the hospital because of abnormal uterine bleeding and pain. Unfortunately, the patient still chose to attempt to maintain her fertility so she refused a hysterectomy even though she had to receive transfusions twice in the last 2 months and could not perform her daily activities and social life.

Psychologically, the pain and frequent admissions to the hospital are also affecting her life, causing her to feel depressed and loose her social life. Adequate counseling provided to her and her husband regarding her condition and the possibility of treatment for pain and infertility may decrease the negative psychological aspects of endometriosis. Support from her family can also increase her self-confidence and help her accept her condition, allowing her to choose the best treatment for her condition.

Since endometriosis is a chronic condition and patients with endometriosis must use medication until menopause, acceptance of the patient's condition is very important because it will increase compliance.

CONCLUSION

This case shows that endometriosis therapy is different for each patient. The biopsychosocial approach is very important for endometriosis patients because the disease affects the patients' daily activities and psychological status. Receiving adequate counseling can improve the patient's acceptance of her condition and improve compliance, which is important because she may require treatment for years until reaching menopause. Moreover, acceptance of her condition can help the patient and her husband choose the best type of treatment.

REFERENCES

[1] Applebaum, G. D.; Iwanczyk, L.; Balingit, P. B. (2004). Endometrioma of the abdominal wall masquerading as hernia. *American Journal of Emergency Medicine*, 22: 621 - 622.

[2] Gourgiotis, S.; Veloudis, G.; Pallas, N.; Lagos, P.; Salemis, N. S.; Villias, C. (2008). Abdominal wall endometriosis: report of two cases. *Romanian Journal of Morphology and Embryology*, 49: 553 - 555.

[3] Hestiantoro, A., Sumapraja, K., Wiweko, B., Pratama, G., Situmorang, H., Kemal, A. (2012). Best practice on IMPERIAL. *Sagung Seto.*

[4] Naftalin, J., Hoo, H., Nunes, N., Holland, T., Mavrelos, D., Jurkovic, D. (2016). Association between ultrasound features of adenomyosis and severity of menstrual pain. *Ultrasound in Obstetrics and Gynecology*, 47:779 - 783.

[5] Campo, S., Campo, V. (2012). Benagiano, G. Infertility and Adenomyosis. *Obstetrics and Gynecology International.*

[6] Tsui, K. H., Lee, W. L., Chen, C. Y., Sheu, B. C., Yen, M. S., Chang, T. C., Wang, P. H. (2014). Medical treatment for adenomyosis and/or adenomyoma. *Taiwan Journal of Obstetric and Gynecology*, 53: 459 - 465.

[7] Myra, J. C., et al. (2011). *Pain Action Alliance to Implement a National Strategy (PAINS)*, issue 6.

[8] Grow, D. R., Filer, R. B. (1991). Treatment of adenomyosis with long-term GnRH analogues: a case report. *Obstetrics and Gynecology*, 78: 538 - 539.

[9] Watkins, K. J., Baldo, T. D. (2004). The infertility experience: Biopsychosocial effects and suggestions for counselors. *Journal of Counseling and Development*, 82: 394 - 402.

[10] Callan, V. J., Hennessey, J. F. (1989). Strategies for coping with infertility. *British Journal of Medical Psychology*, 62: 343 - 354.

[11] Daniels, J. P. (2010). Chronic pelvic pain in woman. *British Medical Journal*, 341: c4834.

In: Obstetric and Gynecology Case Report
Editor: Dwiana Ocviyanti
ISBN: 978-1-53616-711-5

Chapter 17

MULTIDISCIPLINARY APPROACH TO GENDER REASSIGNMENT SURGERY IN A DSD 46XX PATIENT WITH DELAYED DIAGNOSIS OF CONGENITAL ADRENAL HYPERPLASIA: A CASE REPORT

***Kanadi Sumapradja*[1,*], *R. A. Putri*[1], *Achmad Kemal Harzif*[1], *Chaula L. Sukasah*[2] and *Sylvia D. Elvira*[3]**

[1]Department of Obstetrics and Gynecology, Faculty of Medicine, Universitas Indonesia, Dr. Cipto Mangunkusumo Hospital, Jakarta, Indonesia

[2] Department of Surgery, Faculty of Medicine, Universitas Indonesia, Dr. Cipto Mangunkusumo Hospital, Jakarta, Indonesia

[3]Department of Psychiatry, Faculty of Medicine, Universitas Indonesia, Dr. Cipto Mangunkusumo Hospital, Jakarta, Indonesia

[*] Corresponding Author's E-mail: kanadisuma@yahoo.com.

ABSTRACT

The disorder of sex development (DSD) is defined as the congenital conditions in which the development of the chromosomal, gonadal, or anatomical sex is atypical. Congenital adrenal hyperplasia (CAH) consists of a family of disorders caused by reduced activity of enzymes required for the biosynthesis of cortisol in the adrenal cortex, resulting in increased levels of dehydroepiandrosterone sulfate and testosterone. The masculinization of a DSD 46XX patient with CAH is caused by excessive levels of male hormones. During adolescence, the diagnosis of DSD is often an alarming and traumatic event for both the adolescent and the family, considering that this a rare disorder and absolutely foreign to the majority of non-medical individuals. The management of DSD is extraordinarily heterogeneous across centers, and pre- and post-treatment evaluations are mostly subjective, examiner-dependent, and influenced by cultural norms.

In this article, we report a rare case of delayed diagnosis of DSD 46XX in a 23-year-old patient with CAH. The patient exhibiting genital ambiguity and primary amenorrhea, desired to be a male person. The levels of hormones were as follows: high dehydroepiandrosterone sulfate, 937.8μg/dL); high testosterone, 27.3nmL/L; and low estradiol, 45pg/mL, corresponding to the normal levels of a male. A multidisciplinary team, consisting of a reproductive endocrinologist, plastic surgeon, metabolic endocrinologist, psychiatrist, and the hospital ethics committee, collaborated to address the patient's desire regarding her gender condition. Prolonged exposure to androgens results in masculinization of the brain.

Therefore, she preferred to become a male instead of a female. She underwent total laparoscopy hysterectomy and masculinizing reconstructive surgery on her external genitalia.

In addition, prior to and following surgery, the patient received psycho-adaptive therapy.

Keywords: disorder of sex development 46XX, congenital adrenal hyperplasia, gender reassignment surgery, multidisciplinary approach

INTRODUCTION

The disorder of sex Development (DSD) is defined as congenital conditions in which the development of the chromosomal, gonadal, or anatomical sex is atypical. This broad category is divided into three primary groups based on karyotype, namely 46XY; 46XX, and sex chromosome DSD. Secondary groups are formed based on hormonal assessment and imaging [1, 2].

Congenital adrenal hyperplasia (CAH) consists of a family of disorders caused by reduced activity of enzymes required for the biosynthesis of cortisol in the adrenal cortex. The most common defect is 21-hydroxylase (21-OH) deficiency, occurring in 90% of all cases [3]. The disorder appears to be more common in individuals of Hispanic, Slavic, Italian, and European Jewish ancestry. The incidence of genital ambiguity is 1 per 4,500 individuals, though some degree of male under-virilization or female virilization may be present in 2% of live births [4]. In Indonesia, only a limited number of hospitals have a team dedicated for the management of DSD. Thus, currently, data related to DSD remains scarce.

Typically, the management of a DSD patient with CAH depends on the time of diagnosis. In cases in whom CAH is recognized immediately after birth, medical treatment is the treatment of choice. However, in those diagnosed at a later stage of life, it has been suggested to offer the following option to the patients/family: raise the child as a male, postpone the surgery, and suppress puberty until a definitive choice is reached by the patient. Genital surgery continues to be controversial regarding its indications, timing, and technical aspects [5].

During adolescence years, the diagnosis of DSD is often an alarming and traumatic event both for the adolescent and the family, considering that this is a rare disorder and absolutely foreign to the majority of non-medical individuals [6]. The goal of gender reassignment is to improve the quality of life of the patient. The development of the reproductive system, sexual identity, sexual function, and fertility are important factors to be considered in this process [7]. The management of DSD is extraordinarily heterogeneous across centers, and pre- and post-treatment evaluations are mostly subjective, examiner-dependent, and influenced by cultural norms [5].

In this article, we report a rare case of delayed diagnosis of DSD 46XX in a patient with CAH. A multidisciplinary approach was used to address the gender condition of this patient.

Case Report

A 23-year-old patient was referred to our hospital from the Public Hospital in Riau Province due to DSD 46XX. She was delivered by a traditional birth attendant. Initially she was pointed out as a female. During her childhood, she was nurtured as a female.

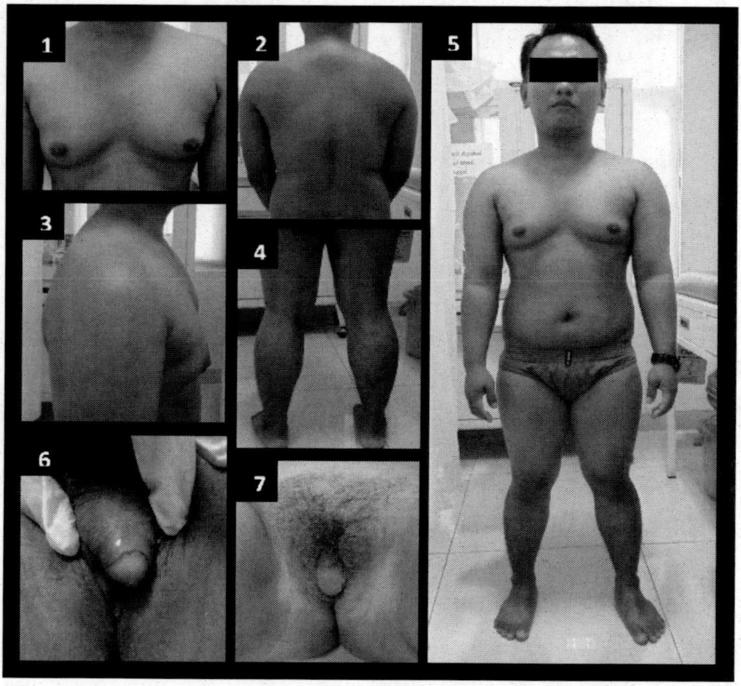

Figure 1. 1) M1 of breast maturity, 2–4 and 7) Ferriman Galleway score >7, 5) male appearance and short stature, 6 and 7) genital ambiguity.

However, after the age of 12 years, her behavior changed dramatically. She began to identify herself as a male individual. Furthermore, her genitals did not resemble those of a normal female. Since she was unable to accept the response from the surrounding, she finally decided to discontinue her education. Initially, her parents recognized a discrepancy in the appearance of her genitals. Unfortunately, they did not have sufficient information to explain the phenomenon, and considered it to be a normal variation. In 2012, the patient was examined by a local urologist and was referred to the Dr. Cipto Mangunkusumo Tertiary Hospital, Jakarta, Indonesia. Unfortunately, her parents postponed this plan due to financial challenges.

The patient is the youngest in a family of seven children who live with their parents. Daily activities include assisting her parents with their work. She performs household chores similar to a male person (i.e., lifts the bucket, fixes the electricity, and paints the wall). Sometimes she is confused regarding her gender, sex, and social identity. Currently, individuals who live in the surrounding call her "Ucok" (a nickname for a young boy). Lately, she began to be attracted to a female, but was unsure how to express her feelings to a woman.

The patient has not experienced menstruation or breast development, and did not report a history of cyclic lower abdominal pain. However, she demonstrates growth of pubic and axillary hair.

Following physical examination, she appeared in good condition and hemodynamically stable. The body mass index of the patient was 27.30kg/m2 (i.e., overweight), while the body height and weight were 148cm and 60kg, respectively. The general status was within normal limits (i.e., no galactorrhea, the Ferriman Galleway score was >7, and the Tanner stage was M1P4).

Gynecological evaluation revealed ambiguous genitalia (i.e., a vagina and phallus of 5cm were observed, without scrotum). Rectovaginal touch showed non-palpable uterus and adnexal mass.

Transrectal ultrasound was performed, and the results were as follows: uterine size 29 × 16 × 26mm, volume 6.72mL, and endometrium 3.7mm, with a regular basal layer.

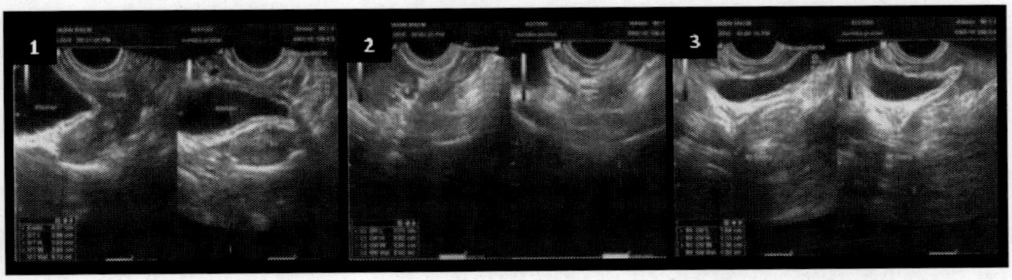

Figure 2. Transrectal ultrasound shows: 1) small uterine size, 2) and 3) small ovaries.

Both ovaries were small (volume of right and left ovaries: 1.32mL and 0.62mL, respectively) with a total number of follicles <6. Computed tomography, previously performed at a different hospital, confirmed the presence of a uterus and absence of testes.

The results of the chromosomal analysis revealed DSD 46XX. Laboratory findings were as follows: normal morning cortisol 8.8μg/dL (normal range, 3.7 – 19.4μg/mL), high dehydroepiandrosterone sulfate (DHEAS) 937.8μg/dL (normal range, 134.2 – 407.4μg/dL), normal anti-mullerian hormone 2.32ng/mL (normal range, 0 – 14.8ng/mL), high testosterone 27.3nmL/L (normal range for male, 4.94 – 32nmol/L), low luteinizing hormone <0.5mIU/mL (normal range for male, 0.57 – 12.07mIU/L), follicle stimulating hormone 2.62mIU/mL (normal range for male, 0.95 – 11.95mIU/mL), estradiol 45pg/mL (normal range for male, 11 – 44pg/mL). The glucose profile was normal in terms of fasting blood glucose, and 1h and 2h glucose tolerance test (89mg/dL, 183mg/dL, and 148mg/dL, respectively). Kidney function was normal in terms of urea and creatinine. The levels of electrolytes were also within normal limits (natrium 138mEq/L, kalium 4.3mEq/L, and chlorine 101.3mEq/L).

The patient was diagnosed with primary amenorrhea, DSD 46XX, ambiguous genitalia, and CAH. A multidisciplinary team, consisting of a reproductive endocrinologist, plastic surgeon, metabolic endocrinologist, psychiatrist, and the ethics committee of the hospital, was formed. An immediate consultation was arranged to assess the case based on every discipline involved in the team.

Examination using abdominal ultrasound did not detect the presence of an adrenal tumor or abnormalities in the abdominal organs. No specific therapy from Metabolic-Endocrine of Internal Medicine. The patient was evaluated by a psychiatrist and diagnosed as follows: axis I, mood adaptation disturbance; axis II, avoidance of personality; axis III, DSD 46XX; axis IV, this medical condition; axis V: current Global Assessment of Functioning score was 80 and the highest level past year was 85. Supportive psychotherapy and psychoeducation for the patient and her family were planned. The plastic surgeon concurred with the initial diagnosis, and planned to perform reconstructive surgery (i.e., radial free forearm flap and implant to enlarge the phallus) to support the gender preference of the patient.

According to a meeting of the multidisciplinary team, the patient identified (i.e., self and gender concept) with the male gender. For preparatory purposes related to the reconstructive surgery, the plastic surgeon reexamined her external genitalia during erection. Considering that the level of testosterone at the time of consultation was already sufficiently high to support her gender identity, the reproductive endocrinologist decided not to administer hormonal support. A member of the ethics committee proposed that the gender reassignment should also proceed legally after the surgery.

She underwent total laparoscopic hysterectomy, performed by a reproductive endocrinologist. The management was continued with the release of cordae and urethroplasty, performed by a plastic surgeon. The decision regarding the hysterectomy was reached based on the patient's request.

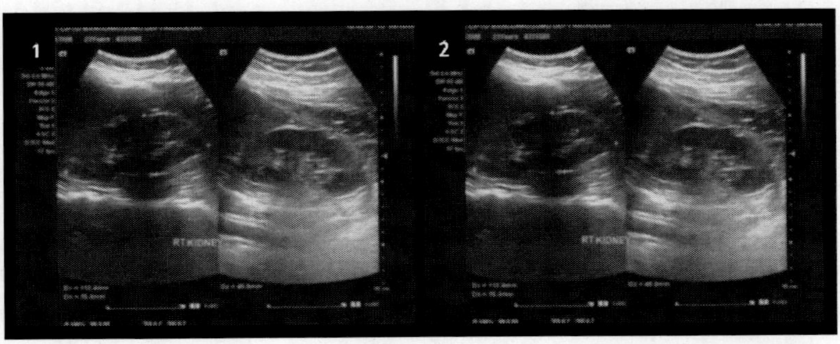

Figure 3. Abdominal ultrasound: Absence of a suprarenal mass.

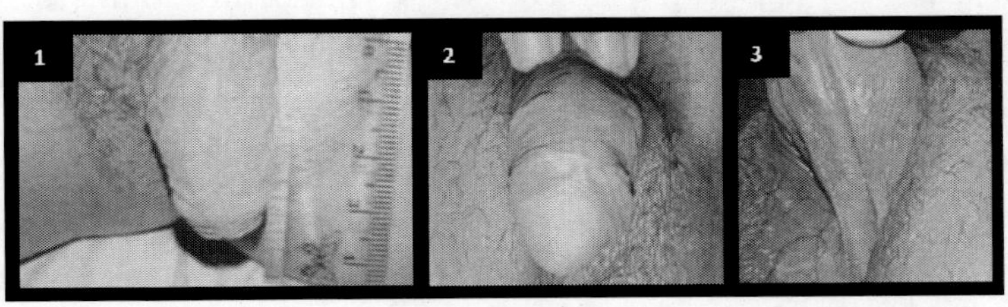

Figure 4. External genitalia in erection condition: 1) penile shaft 4–5 cm, 2) erection position, and 3) cordae.

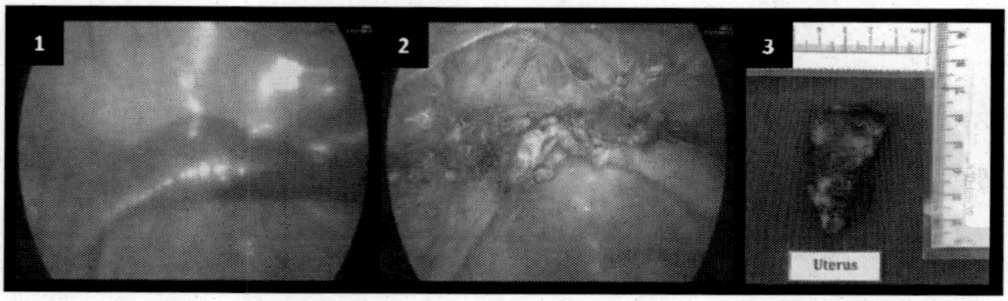

Figure 5. 1 and 2) total laparoscopic hysterectomy, 3) uterus specimen.

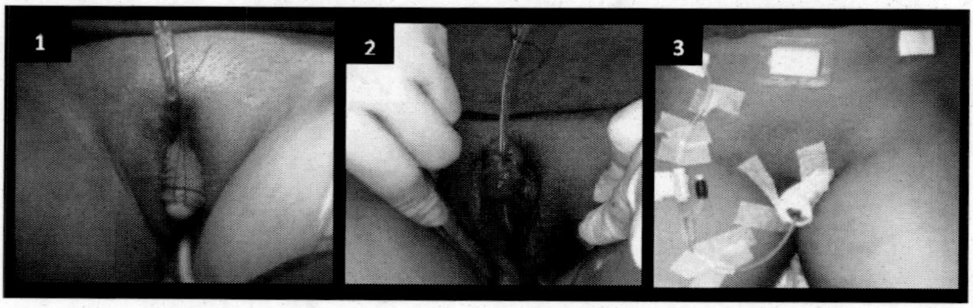

Figure 6. Release of cordae and urethroplasty (step 1), performed by a plastic surgeon.

The psychiatrist administered anti-depressant agents and psycho-supportive therapy. Moreover, the plastic surgeon planned to perform a second procedure (i.e., reconstruction surgery to form the scrotum and phallus) 6 months later.

DISCUSSION

In patients with DSD 46XX, classic CAH represents the most common diagnosis. Usually, there are no gender issues in this group of patients, except in cases of late diagnosis and severe masculinization [5]. In the present case, gender was the main issue due to the delayed diagnosis. The lack of knowledge by the parents and traditional birth attendant regarding genital ambiguity, the minimal information regarding DSD among the community, and financial challenges contributed to this delay. In settings of limited resources, especially in the absence of neonatal screening, examination of the genitalia is crucial for the detection of CAH. Virilization of the external genitalia without palpable gonads should arouse suspicion of

CAH, and is an indication for the urgent referral of the patient to an endocrine specialist [8].

Genital ambiguity can be caused by high exposure to androgens in a 46XX individual, or under-masculinization in a 46XY individual. In 46XX genital ambiguity, the source of high exposure to androgen may be external or internal. Internally, there are two organs responsible for the production of androgens, namely the ovary and adrenal gland [5, 6].

CAH results in increased production of androgens from the adrenal gland due to an enzyme deficiency. The most common defect in CAH is 21-OH deficiency, caused by mutations in the cytochrome CYP21A2 gene. This leads to failure in the synthesis of cortisol due to the impaired conversion of 17α-hydroxyprogesterone to 11-deoxycortisol [9]. Clinical consequences of 21-OH deficiency arise primarily from the overproduction and accumulation of precursors proximal to the blocked enzymatic step. These precursors are shunted into the androgen biosynthesis pathway and further converted to testosterone and dihydrotestosterone [3, 10]. These hormones affect multiple somatic systems that may have psychological implications, including glucose household (at any ages), differentiation of the reproductive tract and presumably the brain (during prenatal development), and growth of primary sex characteristics, development of secondary sex characteristics, further differentiation of the brain, and activation of previously organized brain circuits (during puberty) [11].

Masculinization of patients is observed since childhood. The brain organization theory suggests that, during fetal development, steroid hormones permanently organize the brain in terms of gender, including patterns of sexuality, cognition, temperament, interests, and mental health that are considered "masculine" or "feminine" [12]. In DSD 46XX patients with CAH, prenatal exposure to androgens (the high prenatal levels of male sex hormones to which the genetically female brain is exposed) may shift some, but not all, personality characteristics in the male-typical direction in females [8, 10, 11].

The three components of sexual psychosexual development (i.e., gender identity, gender role, and sexual orientation) may not always be concordant and aligned in individuals with DSD. However, in those with DSD, the primary goal is for gender identity to be consistent with gender assignment [7]. In cases of late diagnosis, it has been suggested to offer the option of raising the child as a boy, and postpone surgery until a definitive choice is reached by the individual. The majority of DSD 46XX patients with CAH are raised as males (usually with a marked degree of genital masculinization) and do not develop gender dysphoria. The cultural environment of the child is of utmost importance in this decision process [5].

As suggested by different studies, the multidisciplinary approach should be established for the management of DSD cases [4]. Such a multidisciplinary team consists of a reproductive endocrinologist, plastic surgeon, psychiatrist, urologist, and ethic-medicolegal consultant. This approach satisfies the requirement to assess and manage DSD patients from different medical perspectives, prior to reaching a consensus based on the preferences of the individual.

As the child develops and reaches adolescence, the gynecologist is again uniquely positioned to assist the family with discussions regarding sexuality and reproductive issues. In addition, many of these conditions are not diagnosed until adolescence when lack of menstruation, pubertal development, or virilization elicits a referral to the gynecologist. Thus, the first physician to diagnose many of these conditions during adolescence may be the gynecologist [2]. The initial evaluation involves assessment of the patient's medical history of familial disorders, a physical examination with particular attention to the genitalia, determination of the karyotype, and (if findings are consistent with CAH) a rapid evaluation of 17-hydroxyprogesterone. However, in Indonesia, finding a laboratory which provides an evaluation of the level of 17-hydroxyprogesterone is challenging. Therefore, initially, the level of total testosterone should be measured to confirm the increased presence of androgens. In cases with high levels of total testosterone, the primary source of androgens should be determined either in the ovary or the adrenal gland by measuring the DHEAS. A high level of DHEAS indicates that the primary source of androgens is the adrenal gland.

Gender is determined by the chromosome, social environment, social role, and sexual orientation. Although the chromosome of this patient was

46XX, the patient's gender identity tended to develop as a male individuals based on the social role, social environment, and sexual orientation [11, 13]. It is truly a great challenge to deal with gender issues in DSD cases. Such research lays the groundwork for additional investigation regarding the contribution of genetic risk, pubertal timing, and sociocultural experience of gender to neural changes underlying mood and anxiety symptoms [14]. Mood conditions, especially depression, anxiety and affective distress, are frequently reported in males and females with CAH. Such conditions may be traced to imbalances of steroid hormones, including cortisol, and the cortisol precursors adrenocorticotropic hormone and corticotropin releasing hormone, a neurotransmitter centrally involved in endocrine, autonomic, immune, and behavioral responses to stress [12]. Psychiatric treatment includes the use of psychopharmacologic agents and supportive psychotherapy techniques [13].

The aims of surgery in DSD patients are as follows: to restore functional genital anatomy allowing future penetrative intercourse (as a male or a female), facilitate future reproduction (as a male or a female) when possible, and reduce urological hazards related to abnormal genitourinary anatomy [5]. For the reconstruction of the genital tubercle in males, surgery is based on the principles of hypospadias surgery, which involves three main steps: (1) degloving of the genital tubercle to assess the severity of the hypospadias based on the level of division of the corpus spongiosum, the degree of hypoplasia of the ventral tissues and the subsequent ventral curvature, the position of the urethral meatus, the length of the urethra to be reconstructed, the size of the genital tubercle, the size and shape of the glans, and the availability of foreskin tissue; (2) refashioning of the missing urethra (i.e., urethroplasty), and (3) refashioning of the penile skin shaft [5].

Although the relevant legislation varies between countries, it is usually allowed to delay a child's gender registration until the medical situation is clarified. Genital surgery continues to be controversial regarding its indications and ethical aspects. The management is extraordinarily heterogeneous across centers, and pre- and post-treatment evaluations are mostly subjective, examiner-dependent, and influenced by cultural norms [5]. The ethical-medicolegal aspect was included in this multidisciplinary team to support the family in processing the legal aspect of gender registration in this patient.

It is important to note that the formation of a multidisciplinary team is more than bringing together different specialists. These specialists create a process for clinical care and decision-making. This process is continuously evaluated and adjusted to optimally serve the patients and the community. It is important that the members of the team communicate with each other on a regular basis to ensure optimal care for the patient and family. Currently, there are many areas for which there are no clear guidelines regarding management. In such cases, the team must reach decisions together with the patient and parents, taking into account a variety of factors (i.e., genetic, endocrine, and anatomic findings) along with the preferences of the individual and the values of the family. Among these decisions, gender reassignment and surgical management are among the most difficult. Thus, communication between the team members regarding their unique perspective, based on their field of expertise, is essential. It has been noted that parents reach different decisions depending on the individual who counsels them regarding surgery. Therefore, it is important for the team members to communicate with the families regarding their different perspectives in an open and caring manner. In addition, the members of the team can discuss all pertinent medical and psychosocial issues prior to the consultation with the family (to ensure a clear understanding of the medical condition), as well as after the consultation (to reach a consensus regarding management) [2].

CONCLUSION

DSD is a clinical condition which requires attention from a clinical perspective, as well as beyond the clinic. Lack of knowledge may significantly contribute to a delayed diagnosis. DSD is a condition that should be managed individually, based on the main needs and values of the patients and their families. Masculinization of the brain and genitalia in patients with delayed diagnosis of DSD 46XX requires a multidisciplinary approach. Raising awareness and advancing knowledge related to genital ambiguity is crucial for the prevention of delayed diagnosis.

REFERENCES

[1] Listyasari, N. A., Santosa, A., Juniarto, A. Z., Faradz, S. M. (2017). Multidisciplinary management of disorders of sex development in indonesia, a prototype for developing country. *Journal of Biomedical and Translational Research,* 01:17 - 22.

[2] Gomez-Lobo, V. (2014). Multidisciplinary care for individuals with disorders of sex development. *Current Opinion in Obstetrics Gynecology,* 26: 366 - 71.

[3] Pang, S., Silverstein, J. (2000). Technical report: congenital adrenal hyperplasia. *Pediatrics,* 106: 1511 - 6.

[4] Chowdhury, M. A. K., Anwar, R.; Saha, A. (2018). Ambiguous genitalia-A social dilemma in Bangladesh: A case report. *International Journal of Surgery Case Reports,* 42: 98 - 101.

[5] Mouriquand, P. D.; Gorduza, D. B.; Gay, C. L.; Meyer-Bahlburg, H. F.; Baker, L.; Baskin, L. S. et al. (2016). Surgery in disorders of sex development (DSD) with a gender issue: If (why), when, and how? *Journal of Pediatric Urology,* 12:139 - 49.

[6] Auchus, R. J., Quint, E. H. (2015). Adolescents with disorders of sex development (DSD)--lost in transition? *Hormone and Metabolic Research,* 47: 367 - 74.

[7] Houk, C. P.; Lee, P. A. (2010). Approach to assigning gender in 46,XX congenital adrenal hyperplasia with male external genitalia: replacing dogmatism with pragmatism. *The Journal of Clinical Endocrinology and Metabolism,* 95: 4501 - 8.

[8] Ganie, Y., Aldous, C., Balakrishna, Y., Wiersma, R. (2018). Congenital adrenal hyperplasia due to 21-hydroxylase deficiency in South Africa. *South African Medical Journal*:108.

[9] Mussig, K.; Kaltenbach, S.; Maser-Gluth, C.; Hartmann, M. F.; Wudy, S. A.; Horger, M. et al. (2006). Late diagnosis of congenital adrenal

hyperplasia due to 21-hydroxylase deficiency. *Experimental and Clinical Endocrinology and Diabetes,* 114: 208 - 14.

[10] Speiser, P. W.; Arlt, W.; Auchus, R. J.; Baskin, L. S.; Conway, G. S.; Merke, D. P. et al. (2018). Congenital adrenal hyperplasia due to steroid 21-hydroxylase deficiency: an endocrine society clinical practice guideline. *The Journal of Clinical Endocrinology and Metabolism,* 103: 4043 - 88.

[11] Meyer- Bahlburg, H. F. (2011). Brain Development and cognitive, psychosocial, and psychiatric functioning in classical 21- hydroxylase deficiency. *Endocr. Dev. Basel Karger,* 20: 88 - 95.

[12] Jordan-Young, R. M. (2012). Hormones, context, and "brain gender": a review of evidence from congenital adrenal hyperplasia. *Social Science and Medicine,* 74:1738 - 44.

[13] Ozbaran, B., Ozen, S., Goksen, D., Korkmaz, O., Onay, H., Cogulu, O. et al. (2013) Psychiatric approaches for disorders of sex development: experience of a multidisciplinary team. *Journal of Clinical Research in Pediatric Endocrinology,* 5: 229 - 35.

[14] Eckstrand, K. L., Travis, M. J., Forbes, E. E., Phillips, M. L. (2016). Sex differences and personalized psychiatric care. *Biological Psychiatry,* 80: e81 - e3.

SECTION 3: GYNECOLOGY

In: Obstetric and Gynecology Case Report ISBN: 978-1-53616-711-5
Editor: Dwiana Ocviyanti

Chapter 18

ONE OF THE MOST RARE GYNECOLOGIC MALIGNANCIES: A SERIAL CASE REPORT ON FALLOPIAN TUBE CANCER

Tofan Widya Utami**, Kade Yudi Saspriyana, Kartiwa Hadi Nuryanto, Hariyono Winarto and Gatot Purwoto

Department of Obstetric and Gynecology, Faculty of Medicine, Universitas Indonesia, Dr. Cipto Mangunkusumo Hospital, Jakarta, Indonesia

ABSTRACT

Fallopian tube cancer (FTC) is one of the most rare malignancies of the female reproductive system, accounting for only 0.14%-1.8% of all gynecologic cancers. Its rarity contributes to the difficulty in making a definite diagnosis and determining its prognosis, and its diagnosis is rarely done preoperatively. The presence of a hydrosalpinx is a hallmark of FTC.

* Corresponding Author's E-mail: tofanwidya@yahoo.com.

Here, we report three cases of FTC to explore an approach for its diagnosis and management. Because FTC shares similar clinical findings with ovarian carcinoma, it is often diagnosed intraoperatively. The elevation of serum CA125 levels contributes to the diagnosis of FTC. Surgical cytoreduction followed by chemotherapy is the best therapeutic option for FTC.

Keywords: fallopian tube cancer, diagnosis, management

INTRODUCTION

Fallopian tube cancer (FTC) is one of the most rare malignancies of the female reproductive system, accounting for only 0.14%-1.8% of all gynecologic cancers. Preoperative diagnosis of FTC is difficult because its clinical and histological findings are similar to those of ovarian carcinoma [1]. However, several studies have reported that 40%-60% of high-grade serous carcinomas that have been classified as ovarian carcinomas actually originate from the fallopian tubes [2]. For the initial management of FTC, primary surgery is preferred followed by systemic chemotherapy.

Here, we report three cases of FTC to explore an approach for its diagnosis and management.

CASE REPORT

Case 1

A 54-year-old unmarried woman presented to our oncology clinic with nausea, vomiting, and abdominal pain experienced since 1 month prior to admission. She experienced no vaginal bleeding or difficulty in micturition and defecation. Her vital signs were stable and the Eastern Cooperative Oncology Group (ECOG) performance status was 0. Pelvic examination revealed a moderate amount of free fluid in the abdominopelvic cavity. Chest X-rays showed the presence of infiltrates in both lungs and suspected left pleural effusion. Abdominal computed tomography (CT) showed an enhancedleft adnexal lesion, omental cake, ascites, and adhesive small bowel obstruction, with the possibility of primary ovarian malignancy. The patient's serum CA125 level was elevated at 1250 U/ml (normal value: 0-35 U/ml). She underwent exploratory laparotomy with the following findings: approximately 2000cc ascites, normal uterus, normal ovaries, enlargement of the right fallopian tube (diameter, 5 × 1 cm), and enlargement of the left fallopian tube (5 × 1.5 cm). Both fallopian tubes were adhered to the rectosigmoid. The operative procedures used included total hysterectomy, bilateral salpingo-oophorectomy, omentectomy, peritoneal biopsy, and sigmoid loop colostomy due to severe adhesion between the lesion and sigmoid colon. Pathological analyses revealed oorly differentiated metastatic adenocarcinoma in theomentum and peritoneum, and the uterus and adnexa showed high-grade serous carcinoma that was found in both ovaries and fallopian tubes. Cytological analyses of the pleural effusion fluid showed positive results for tumor metastases. Sixes cycles of docetaxel-carboplatin chemotherapy wereadministered from February to June 2018. Clinical evaluation conducted following the sixth cycle of chemotherapy did not reveal any residual mass based on physical examination. Further, abdominal CT revealed that there was no residual mass in the pelvic cavity, minimal fluid collection in the pouch of Douglas, hepatomegaly with multiple nodules in the fourth segment of liver, and minimal left pleural effusion. The CA125 level (24.8 U/mL) reduced within the normal limit (0-35 U/mL).

Case 2

A 47-year-old woman (parity 3) presented to our oncology clinic with a lower abdominal mass that was present since the past year. She experienced no abdominal pain, vaginal bleeding, and difficulty in micturition and defecation. She had never used contraception. At presentation, her vital signs were stable and the ECOG performance status was 0. Pelvic examination revealed a 16-cm non-tender, mobile adnexal mass and normal uterus.

Ultrasound examination revealed a septatedcystic mass with a solid portion, sized 100 × 59 × 138 mm, with low-resistance blood flow in the solid portion (resistance index = 0.19), corresponding to a bilateral cystic ovarian neoplasm withsuspected malignancy (Figure 1). Abdominal CT revealed a lobulated cystic mass (13.5 × 11.8 × 7.6 cm) with septation and papillary projections on the left adnexa. The mass was suspected to be adhered to the rectum, bladder, and uterus, suggestive of malignancy. Uterus appeared normal, andno lymphadenopathy or intra-abdominal metastasis was observed. However, the serum CA125 level had increased (360.5 U/mL). Therefore, the patient underwent laparotomy for the assessment of the suspected malignant ovarian neoplasm.

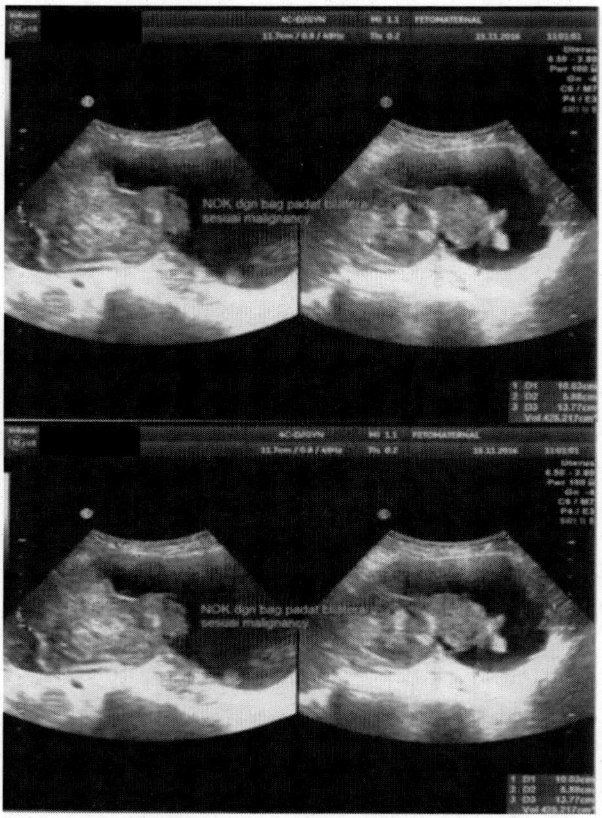

Figure 1. Bilateral cystic adnexal mass with a solid portion and low-resistance neovascularization on ultrasound.

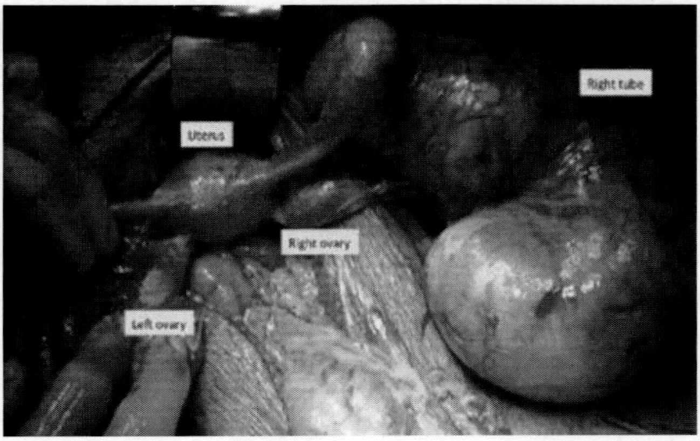

Figure 2. Intraoperative findings of a normal uterus and both ovaries and enlargement of both fallopian tubes.

Intraoperatively, we found a cystic/solid mass with a smooth surface and no adhesions sized 20 × 10 × 10 cm from the right fallopian tube and sized 10 × 2 × 2 cm from the left fallopian tube. The uterus and both ovaries were within normal limits (Figure 2), with no ascites. We performed bilateral salpingectomy and sent the specimens for frozen section examinationthat revealed right FTC and atypical cells in the left fallopian tube. The procedure was continued with complete surgical staging (total hysterectomy, bilateral oophorectomy, pelvic and para-aortic lymphadenectomy, and omentectomy). Paraffin block sectioning revealed high-grade serous carcinoma of the right fallopian tube and a left paratubal cyst. There were no tumor masses on the omentum, peritoneum, uterus, and all pelvic and para-aortic lymph nodes. Therefore, the patient was diagnosed with stage IA high-grade primary FTC. The patient received six cycles of chemotherapy with carboplatin and paclitaxel at intervals of 3 weeks. She was declared clinically disease free 8 months thereafter.

Case 3

A 51-year-old postmenopausal woman (parity 0) was admitted for vaginal discharge persisting for 1 month. Per speculum examination showed serosanguinous discharge and smooth cervix and vagina. Vaginal examination revealed a normal sized anteverted uterus with clear fornices and no palpable mass on both adnexa. Further, ultrasound examination showed right and left hydrosalping sized 7 × 3 cm, with a 3.6- × 2.2-cm intraluminal mass (color score = 3). Both ovaries were normal. There were multiple leiomyomas of the uterus and no ascites (Figure 3). The serum CA125 level was normal at 11.5 U/ml. The patient was suspected of having FTC and underwent laparotomy. Intraoperatively, we found that the uterus was enlarged with multiple uterine fibroids andenlarged fallopian tubes (4 × 2 × 1 and 4 × 2 × 2 cm). The presence ofascites was not noted, and both ovaries were within normal limits (Figure 4). We performed laparotomy with total hysterectomy and bilateral salpingo ophorectomy and sent the specimensfor frozen sectioning. The frozen sections revealed adenocarcinoma of both fallopian tubes. The procedure was continued with complete surgical staging (total hysterectomy, pelvic and para-aortic lymphadenectomy, omentectomy, appendectomy, and peritoneal biopsy). Paraffin block sectioning revealed high-grade serous carcinoma of both fallopian tubes. The patient was diagnosed with stage IB high-grade primary FTC, and adjuvant chemotherapy with carboplatin and paclitaxel was planned.

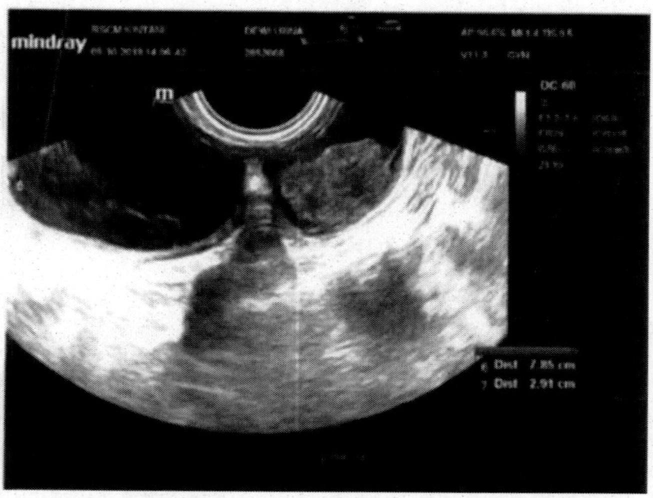

Figure 3. Left hydrosalping with an intraluminal mass.

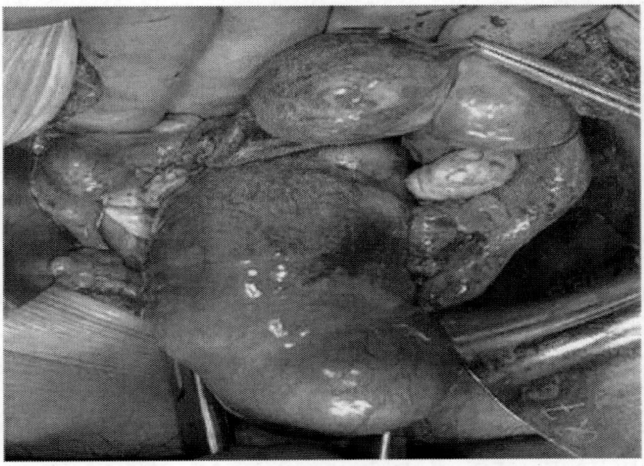

Figure 4. Intraoperative findings of multiple uterine fibroids and enlargement of both fallopian tubes.

Informed consent has been obtained from all patients involved in this study.

Discussion

Epithelial carcinomas of ovarian, fallopian tube, and peritoneal origin show similar clinical characteristics and behavior. Primary FTC is rarely seen clinically due to hidden lesions and availability of minimal preoperative screening methods as well as limited cases and clinical experience, with most cases being found accidentally during operations [3]. Due to its rarity, we presented three cases to explore the diagnosis and management of FTC.

Kurman and Shih (2010) reported that serous ovarian tumors arise from the implantation of epithelium (benign or malignant) from the fallopian tubes [4]. Because the fallopian tubes are situated very close to the ovaries and uterus, the identification of primary lesions in patients with advanced carcinoma is sometimes difficult. In patients with FTC, although there may be no abnormalities in the ovaries and endometrium, there may be metastasis due to lymphatic communication. The size of the tumor of the fallopian tube is bigger than those ofthe ovaries and endometrium [3].

FTC is commonly found in women aged 40-60 years. Its symptoms include abdominopelvic pain, pressure, and vaginal bleeding. Latzko's triad of symptoms comprising intermittent, profuse, serosanguinous vaginal discharge; colicky abdominal pain relieved by discharge; and an abdominal or pelvic mass have been reported in 15% of FTC cases [5]. Because the clinical manifestations of FTC are somewhat heterogeneous (e.g., abdominal pain and abdominal enlargement, as observed in our cases) and the incidence rate is extremely low, the preoperative misdiagnosis rate is high. Baekelandt et al. reported only 2% correct preoperative diagnosis of FTC, whereas Meng et al. reported that up to 50% of patients were intraoperatively misdiagnosed [6].

The serum CA125 level is essential for FTC diagnosis and follow-up, with elevated levels reported in 65% of FTC cases. Fallopian tube carcinoma characteristically appears as a fusiform swelling that may have the external appearance of a hydrosalpinx or hematosalpinx [7]. Some studies have reported that CA125 is expressed by PFTC10, and it was found to be elevated atthe pretreatment stage, which correlated well with the disease stage [8].

There are several imaging modalitiesused for suspected gynecologic malignancies including ultrasound, CT, and magnetic resonance imaging (MRI). CT and MRI may show the appearance of a small, solid, and lobulated mass. Furthermore, a solid papillary intratubal mass can be used for predicting FTC [9]. MRI features that differentiate fallopian tube carcinoma from ovarian carcinoma include the presence of hydrosalpinges and intrauterine fluid accumulation [10].

Surgery is the treatment of choice for FTC. For late-stage FTC, primary surgical cytoreduction followed by systemic chemotherapy due to lymphatic and hematogenous spread is preferred [11].

The failure to perform an optimal cytoreduction may be caused by technical problems or related to the poor performance status of the patient, e.g., additional abdominal or retroperitoneal disease, large-bulk of tumor, bulky disease in the porta hepatis region, bowel involvement, parenchymal liver involvement, presence of ascites, and patient's ability to tolerate cytoreduction.

Chemotherapy is usually initiated within 2-4 weeks of surgery as soon as itis feasible. However, limited data are availablesupporting the fact that a delay of more than a month in instituting chemotherapy may result in a poorer outcome. For first-line chemotherapy for FTC, the standard IV regimen uses a platinum agent and taxanes. Carboplatin is preferred over cisplatin because multiple trials have consistently demonstrated that carboplatin is better tolerated and causes fewer non-hematologic side effects [12].

CONCLUSION

Primary FTC is a rare gynecologic malignancy. Its diagnosis is rarely made preoperatively because of its similarities to ovarian carcinoma, although the treatment is similar. Surgical cytoreduction followed by chemotherapy remains the best therapeutic option for this malignancy.

REFERENCES

[1] Kanimozhi, G., Kotasthane, D. and Koteeswaran, G. (2012). A case report of fallopian tubal carcinoma. *The Internet Journal of Pathology*, 13 (2).

[2] Berek, J. S., Crum, C., and Friedlander, M. (2015). Cancer of the ovary, fallopian tube, and peritoneum. *International Journal of Gynecology & Obstetrics*, 131 (Suppl. 2): S111-S122.

[3] Ma, Y. and Duan, W. (2014). Clinical and survival analysis of 36 cases of primary fallopian tube carcinoma. *World Journal of Surgical Oncology*, 12: 311.

[4] Nanaiah, S. P., Rathod, P. S., Rajkumar, N. N., Kundargi, R., Subbian, A., Ramachandra, P. V., Krishnappa, S., Narayan, A., Devi, U. K. and Uttamchand, B. D. (2014). Primary carcinoma of the fallopian tube: a

review of a single institution experience of 8 cases. *The Scientific World Journal*, 2014: 630731.

[5] Navin Noushad, S. and Suresh Kumar D. (2016). Primary fallopian tube cancer: a rare gynecological malignancy. *American Journal of Cancer Case Reports*, 4: 129-133.

[6] Pectasides, D., Pectasides, E. and Economopoulos, T. (2006). Fallopian tube carcinoma: a review. *Oncologist*, 11: 902-9112.

[7] Jaison, J., Katre, R. and Joshi, S. (2017). Primary fallopian tube carcinoma: a case report. *MIMER Medical Journal*, 1: 34-36.

[8] Pandey, D., Bhalla, V., Mittal, A. and Shetty, J. (2015). Primary fallopian tube cancer in the setting of endometriosis. *International Journal of Reproduction, Contraception, Obstetrics and Gynecology*, 4: 1571-1573.

[9] Rexhepi, M., Trajkovska, E., Ismaili, H., Besimi, F. and Rufati, N. (2017). Primary fallopian tube carcinoma: a case report and literature review. *Open Access Macedonian Journal of Medical Sciences*, 5: 344-348.

[10] Winarto, H. and Fernando, D. (2017). Identifying features of primary fallopian tube carcinoma using magnetic resonance imaging. *International Medical Case Reports Journal*, 10: 213-217.

[11] Boufettal, H. and Samouh, N. (2014). Primary fallopian tube carcinoma: a case report. *The Pan African Medical Journal*, 18: 263.

[12] Sama, A. R., and Schilder, R. J. (2014). Refractory fallopian tube carcinoma - current perspectives in pathogenesis and management. *International Journal of Women's Health*, 6: 149-157.

In: Obstetric and Gynecology Case Report ISBN: 978-1-53616-711-5
Editor: Dwiana Ocviyanti

Chapter 19

FALLOPIAN TUBE CARCINOMA: A CASE REPORT ON ITS HISTOPATHOLOGICAL ASPECT

***Tofan Widya Utami*[1,*], *Kade Yudi Saspriyana*[1], *Hartono Tjahjadi*[2] *and Kartiwa Hadi Nuryanto*[1]**

[1]Gynecology Oncology Division, Department of Obstetric and Gynecology, Faculty of Medicine, Universitas Indonesia, Dr. Cipto Mangunkusumo Hospital, Jakarta, Indonesia

[2]Department of Pathology Anatomy, Faculty of Medicine, Universitas Indonesia, Dr. Cipto Mangunkusumo Hospital, Jakarta, Indonesia

ABSTRACT

Fallopian tube carcinoma (FTC) is one of the rarest malignancies of female reproductive system, accounting for only 0.14%-1.8% of all gynecological cancers. Establishing a clear diagnosis and prognosis of FTC are generally considered difficult. In this study, we aimed to determine the

[*] Corresponding Author's E-mail: tofanwidya@yahoo.com.

histopathology of FTC and to determine the correlation between its histopathological and clinical findings. A 54-year-old unmarried woman presented with nausea, vomiting, and abdominal pain since 1 month prior to admission. She was diagnosed with suspected ovarian carcinoma with pleural effusions based on clinical and tumor marker tests and imaging. Accordingly, exploratory laparotomy was performed, and ascites and enlarged fallopian tubes that adhered to the rectosigmoid were noted. Subsequently, she underwent total hysterectomy, bilateral salpingo-oophorectomy, omentectomy, peritoneal biopsy, and loop sigmoid colostomy because of the adhesion. Pathological analysis revealed high-grade serous carcinoma in both fallopian tubes and ovaries. Furthermore, pleural fluid cytology showed positive results for a metastatic tumor. Thus, six cycles of docetaxel-carboplatin chemotherapy were administered. Primary FTC is a rare gynecological malignancy. Serous FTC resembles the tumors of its ovarian counterparts with papillae, cellular buds, slit-like glandular spaces, solid sheets, and occasionally tumor giant cells and psammoma bodies.

Keywords: fallopian tube carcinoma, histopathology

INTRODUCTION

Fallopian tube carcinoma (FTC) is one of the rarest malignancies of the female reproductive system, accounting for only 0.14%-1.8% of all gynecological cancers. Its histological and clinical findings are similar to those of ovarian carcinoma, and, as such, a preoperative diagnosis of FTC is clinically difficult to establish [1]. Nonetheless, several studies have reported that 40%-60% of high-grade serous carcinomas classified as ovarian carcinomas essentially originated from the fallopian tubes [2]. Although the reported incidence of several microscopic subtypes of invasive FTC considerably varies, 70%, 10%, and 20% cases are of serous, endometrioid, and other types of FTC, respectively [3].

Primary fallopian tube carcinoma is rarely seen clinically due to hidden lesions, an absence of recommended screening methods, and relatively limited clinical experience, to the extent that a number of cases have been accidentally detected during other gynecological surgeries. Intraluminal tubal fluid can be discharged through the uterus-vagina route when fimbria atresia occurs, and this is usually found in early cases. In case of an open fimbrial end, the tumor cells would come into the abdominal cavity where they could easily grow, and this is found mostly in advanced cases, where the prognosis is rather poor [4].

CASE DESCRIPTION

A 54-year-old unmarried woman presented with nausea, vomiting, and abdominal pain since 1 month prior to admission at our oncology clinic. Neither vaginal bleeding nor difficulty in micturition and defecation was noted. Her vital signs were stable, and the ECOG performance status score was 0. Pelvic examination revealed a moderate amount of abdominal/pelvic free fluid. Bilateral pulmonary infiltrates and suspected left pleural effusion were observed on chest X-ray. In addition, abdominal CT showed left adnexal lesion with enhancement, omental cake, ascites, and adhesive small bowel obstruction with possible primary ovarian malignancy, and the CA-125 level was 1250 U/mL. She underwent exploratory laparotomy, and during the operation, the following were found: ascitic fluid (approximately 2,000 mL), normal uterus and ovaries, and enlarged right (diameter, 5 × 1 cm) and left (diameter, 5 × 1.5 cm) fallopian tubes that adhered to the rectosigmoid. Subsequently, total hysterectomy, bilateral salpingo-oophorectomy, omentectomy, peritoneal biopsy, and loop sigmoid colostomy (because of severe adhesion between the mass and sigmoid) were performed. Pathological analyses revealed the omentum and peritoneum were poorly differentiated metastatic of adenocarcinomas (Figure 5), its adnexa had high-grade serous carcinoma found in both ovaries and fallopian tubes (Figure 1, 2, 3, 4), its uterine subserous had metastatic adenocarcinomas. The result of pleural fluid cytology was positive for a metastatic tumor. Thus, docetaxel-carboplatin chemotherapy was administered for six cycles from February to June 2018. After this treatment, no residual mass was noted on physical examination. In addition, abdominal CT showed the absence of a residual mass in the pelvic cavity, minimal fluid collection in the pouch of Douglas, hepatomegaly with multiple nodules in the fourth liver segment, and minimal left pleural effusion. The CA-125 level was 24.8 U/mL.

Discussion

Epithelial carcinomas of ovarian, fallopian tube, and peritoneal origin show similar clinical characteristics and behaviors. Primary FTC is rarely observed clinically because of hidden lesions, inadequate preoperative screening methods, and limited cases and clinical experiences. In fact, most cases have been discovered accidentally during operation [4].

Kanimozhi, et al. (2012) reported that serous tumors arise from the implantation of epithelium (benign or malignant) from the fallopian tube [1]. The fallopian tubes connect the ovaries to the uterus, and because these organs are intertwined, sometimes difficult identifying primary lesions in advanced stage. In patients with FTC, the ovaries and endometrium may have no abnormalities, but metastatic lymph nodes may be present. Additionally, the tumor sizes in the fallopian tubes are larger than those in the ovaries and endometrium [4-6].

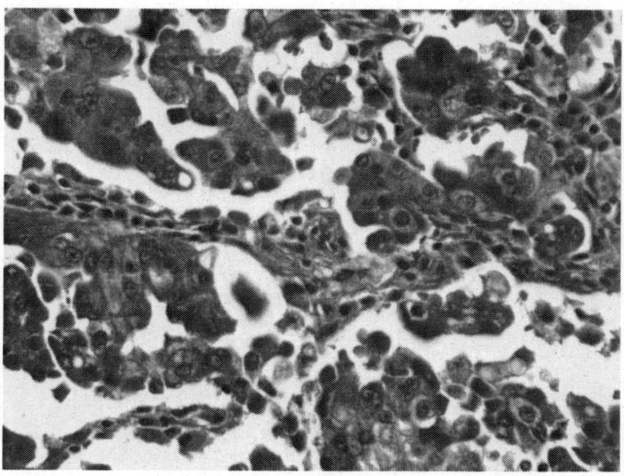

Figure 1. Left ovary. An infiltrative tumor was present in the ovarian parenchyma, and the tumor cells were pleomorphic with coarse chromatin and eosinophilic cytoplasm (Mitoses > 12/10 HPF).

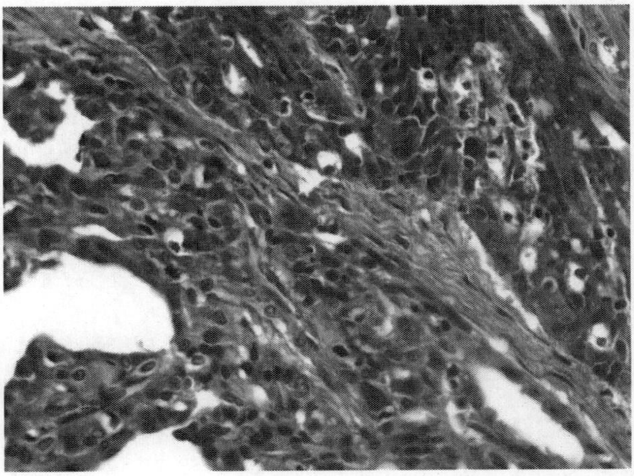

Figure 2. Right ovary. Cystic formation with papillary and tumor growth was observed in the lymph area.

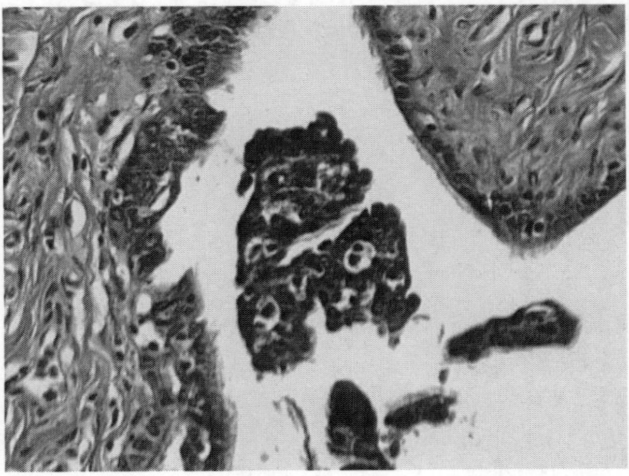

Figure 3. Left fallopian tube. Transition from normal simple epithelia to epithelial dysplasia, carcinoma *in situ*, and early invasive carcinoma were noted.

Regarding gross features of FTC, 3%-13% of cases is bilaterality, and the average tumor size is 5 cm. The fallopian tubes are dilated in over 50% of cases, which intraoperatively can be mistaken for a hydrosalpinx, hematosalpinx, or pyosalpinx. The tumor can appear as ≥1 yellow to tan nodules or a mass that fills the tubal lumen. Hemorrhage or necrosis is frequent. A small percentage of tumors are located at the fimbriated end [6-8].

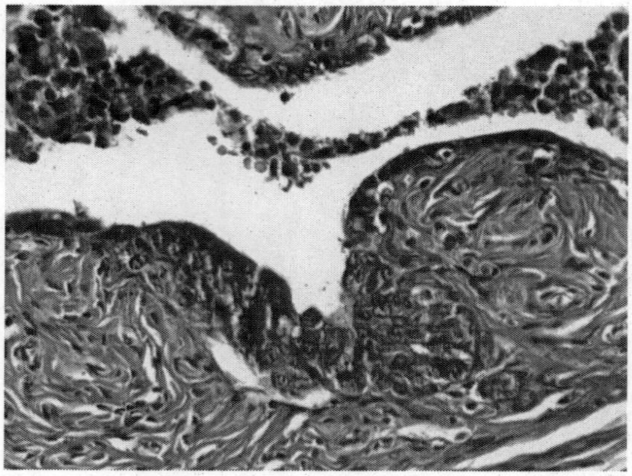

Figure 4. Right fallopian tube. Transition from normal simple epithelia to stratified epithelia and small cell tumor in the luminal area between the plicae were noted.

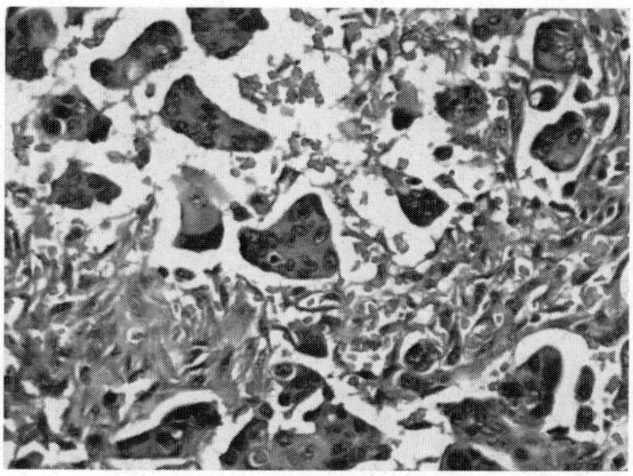

Figure 5. Omentum. Malignant epithelial tumor with a glandular structure and solid sheet was observed. The tumor cells were pleomorphic with vesicular and hyperchromatic nuclei and eosinophilic cytoplasm.

Fallopian Tube Carcinoma is the earliest morphologically recognizable form of carcinoma. Absence of the invasion of the underlying tubal stroma and presence of cytological abnormalities that result in the fallopian tube epithelium appearing darker than the adjacent normal epithelium under low-power magnification are typical for FTC. In cases with invasive carcinoma in the same tube, FTC may be found directly adjacent to the invasion and occur to be unifocal or multifocal [3]. The luminal border may be straight or exhibit variable amounts of irregular contours and hobnail morphology.

Small tufts of detached cells can be found within the tubal lumen, increased with stratification. The lesional cells are seen to lack cilia and show variable combinations of nuclear enlargement, increased nuclear-to-cytoplasmic ratio, hyperchromasia or irregular chromatin distribution, polarity loss, prominent nucleoli, and mitotic figures [8].

The lesional cells of tubal invasive carcinomas show secretory cell differentiation. In addition, they cytologically resemble the cells of high-grade serous carcinoma. Most FTC should be considered as being of serous histological type, because there is pathogenic relationship between FTC and invasive high-grade serous carcinoma. Therefore we should use the diagnostic terms "serous tubal intraepithelial carcinoma" and "tubal intraepithelial carcinoma" as a synonymous terminology. High-grade serous carcinomas within the lumen of the fallopian tubes may be small without enlargement of the tubes and lack the invasion of the underlying tubal stroma. Such morphology in occasional cases can overlap with the upper morphologic limit of TIC, especially when the latter shows an increased degree of stratification. In such cases, the diagnostic threshold between TIC and a small intraluminal high-grade serous carcinoma without the invasion of the underlying tubal stroma is subjective, with varying opinions among authors [8].

CONCLUSION

Primary FTC is a rare gynecological malignancy. Serous FTC resembles its ovarian carcinoma counterparts, with papillae, cellular buds, slit-like glandular spaces, solid sheets, and occasionally tumor giant cells and psammoma bodies. Most of them are high grade, and necrosis and vascular space invasion are common.

Conflict of Interest Statement: The authors declare no conflict of interest in preparing this article.

Funding: The authors received no specific grant from any funding agency in the public, commercial, or not-for-profit sectors.

REFERENCES

[1] Kanimozhi, G., Kotasthane, D., Kotesswaran, G., (2012). A case report of fallopian tubal carcinoma. *The Internet Journal of Pathology*: 13.

[2] Berek, J. S., Crum, C., Friedlander, M., (2015). Cancer of the ovary, fallopian tube, and peritoneum. *Int. J. Gynacel. Obstet,* 131: S111-S122.

[3] Clement, P. B., & Young, R. H., (2013). The fallopian tube and broad ligament. In: Clement, P. B., & Young, R. H. (Eds), *Atlas of gynecologic surgical pathology,* Elsevier: 299-321

[4] Ma, Y., Duan, W., (2014). Clinical and survival analysis of 36 cases of primary fallopian tube carcinoma. *World J. Surg. Oncol,* 12: 311.

[5] Nanaiah, S. P., Rathod, P. S., Rajkumar, N. N., Kundargi, R., Subbian, A., Ramachandra, P. V., Krishnappa, S., Narayan, A., Devi, U. K., Uttamchand, B. D., (2014). Primary carcinoma of the fallopian tube: a review of a single institution experience of 8 cases. *Scientific World Journal,* 630731.

[6] Pectasides, D., Pectasides, E., Economopoulos, T., (2006). Fallopian tube carcinoma: a review. *Oncologist,* 11: 902-912.

[7] Rexhepi, M., Trajkovska, E., Ismaili, H., Besimi, F., Rufati, N., (2017). Primary fallopian tube carcinoma: A case report and literature review. *Open Access Maced. J. Med. Sci,* 5: 344-348.

[8] Vang, R., & Wheeler, J. E., (2011). Diseases of the fallopian tube and paratubal region. In: Kurman, R. J., Ronnett, B. M., & Ellenson, L. R. (Eds). *Blaustein's pathology of the female genital tract,* Springer, 6th edition: 530-572.

In: Obstetric and Gynecology Case Report
Editor: Dwiana Ocviyanti
ISBN: 978-1-53616-711-5

Chapter 20

APPROACH AND MANAGEMENT OF CERVICAL FIBROIDS: A CASE REPORT

Eka Rusdianto Gunardi and Hesti Nurmala Rizqi*

Department of Obstetric and Gynecology, Faculty of Medicine, Universitas Indonesia, Dr. Cipto Mangunkusumo Hospital, Jakarta, Indonesia

ABSTRACT

Cervical fibroids are one of the most interesting findings in fibroid cases owing to their location relative to other important structures. In cases involving a large cervical fibroid, the symptoms are mostly related to anterior and posterior mechanical pressures from the fibroid. Thus, the management should be aimed at releasing these pressures by removing the mass through myomectomy or hysterectomy. Considering the high risk of bladder and bowel injury, these procedures should be precisely performed with advanced understanding of anatomical alterations related to the fibroid. We report a case of a large cervical fibroid in a patient with a history of laparotomy exploration. In this case, we were unable to perform hysterectomy due to severe adhesion. The patient was a 40-year-old female

* Corresponding Author's E-mail: eka_dhikita@yahoo.co.id.

with concomitant endometriosis. Subsequently, a gonadotropin-releasing hormone agonist was administered and the patient was referred to our hospital. We performed relaparotomy hysterectomy, and the cervical fibroid was completely removed. Notably, the bladder and bowel remained intact without other complications.

Keywords: cervical fibroid, cervical myoma, leiomyoma, hysterectomy, myomectomy

INTRODUCTION

Uterine fibroids are the most common benign tumors observed in females. Their prevalence is related to the reproductive cycle, with increased prevalence in females of reproductive age. Of note, thus far, the presence of a uterine fibroid before puberty has not been reported. However, it is observed in >70% of females who have undergone hysterectomy [1, 2]. Fortunately, most of the fibroids are asymptomatic, and the symptoms are variable depending on the location and size of fibroids. Uterine fibroids are usually found in the uterine corpus, especially intramural fibroids. One of the most challenging types of fibroids is cervical fibroid, accounting for 1% – 2% of all uterine fibroid cases. In patients in whom the fibroid is anteriorly located, the mass may push the bladder and urethra, leading to voiding dysfunction, either retention or frequency [1-5].

CASE REPORT

A 40-year-old female was referred from a Level 2 hospital to our hospital. She complained of abdominal enlargement initially observed 3 years prior to admission. In 2016, she visited Tiara Sella Hospital (Bengkulu, Indonesia) and was scheduled to undergo surgery. However, at that time, it was difficult to perform the surgery due to severe adhesion. To control the disease, the treating physician administered a gonadotropin-releasing hormone agonist for 4 months and referred the patient to a Level 3 hospital. Currently, the patient has no complaints of heavy bleeding, micturition problems, or dysmenorrhea.

Physical examination revealed that the uterus could be palpated between the umbilicus and symphysis.

Following speculum examination, we observed bulging of the anterior cervix. However, it was not possible to visualize the portio due to the distortion caused by the mass. According to ultrasound examination, the presence of a mass with well-defined borders (size: 88 × 84 × 62mm) was revealed at the basal part of the uterus, specifically at the anterior corpus, which appeared to be a cervical fibroid. In addition, we identified two cystic masses (size: 34 × 30 and 25 × 25mm) at both adnexa, which were suspected to be bilateral endometriosis cysts.

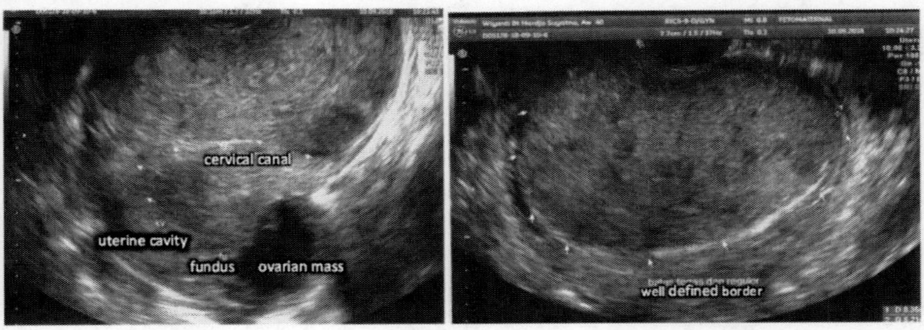

Figure 1. Ultrasound examination of the cervical fibroid.

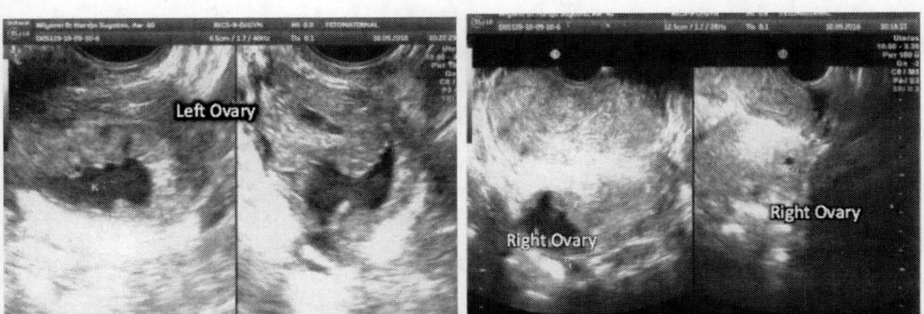

Figure 2. Ultrasound examination: The right and left adnexa.

The patient was surgically treated, and adhesion was found among the peritoneum, bowel, and uterus. Moreover, we found cystic masses on both ovaries. While performing adhesiolysis, the cystic masses were ruptured, releasing a brown fluid. Subsequently, we removed the mass located on the anterior cervix.

Further, we performed hysterectomy. In brief, after the uterine arteries were clamped, cut, and sutured, we proceeded to detach the posterior part. We performed traction to expose the uterosacral ligaments. Subsequently, the ligaments were clamped, cut, and sutured. We identified the posterior part of the vagina, incised the posterior fornix, and cut the lateral side along the junction of the vagina and portio until we reached the anterior vagina. We identified the cervical fibroid (size: 11 × 8 × 6cm), which was anteriorly located. After separating the uterus from the surrounding tissues, it was possible to remove the uterus with the fibroid.

The specimen was histopathologically examined, and the results confirmed that the mass was a mesenchymal tumor with well-defined borders comprising smooth muscle cells with irregular fiber, tumor cell, with uniform shape, and eosinophilic cytoplasm. No mitosis was found as we diagnosed the tumor to be a cervical fibroid. Other notable findings included an endometrial stroma and gland extending into the myometrium of the uterine corpus. These findings correspond to those of adenomyosis at the uterine corpus.

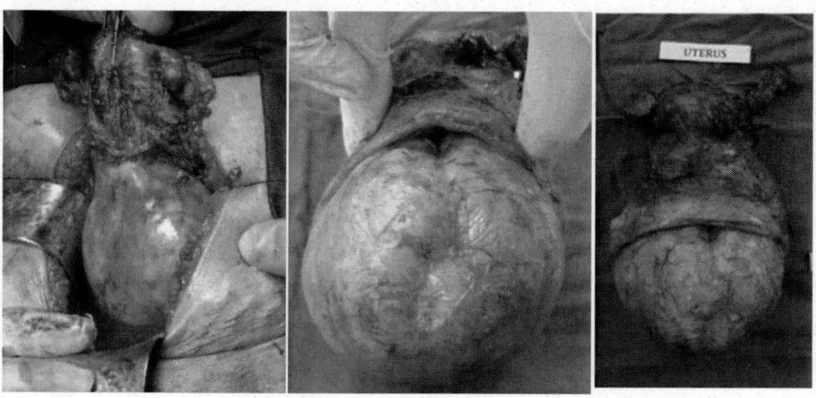

Figure 3. Cervical fibroid.

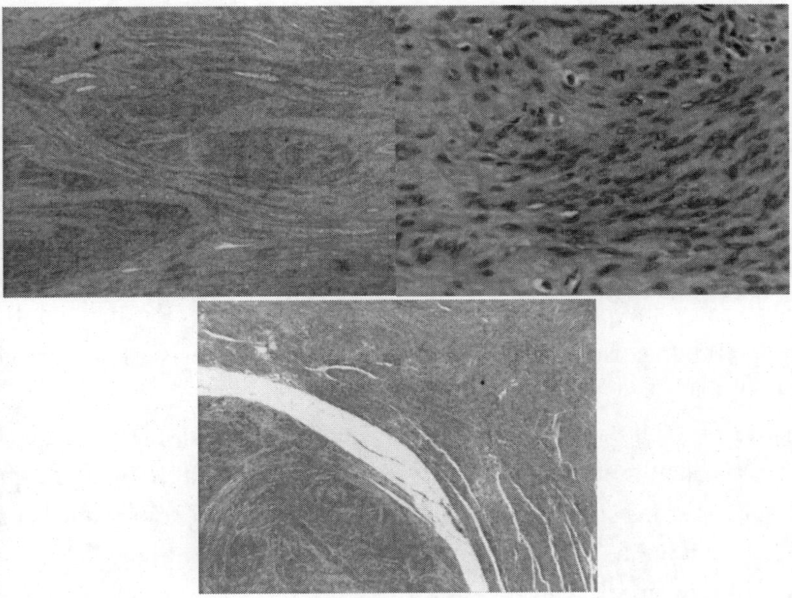

Figure 4. Histopathological results.

DISCUSSION

The cervix is one the most distal parts of the uterus comprising collagen and fibromuscular tissues. In response to dysregulation of smooth muscles, the cells proliferate, resulting in the development of a benign tumor (i.e., a fibroid). Small cervical fibroids may be asymptomatic; however, large cervical fibroids may anteriorly push the bladder and cause voiding problems or posteriorly obstruct the rectum [6, 7]. In the present case, despite its large size, the fibroid did not interfere with micturition or defecation in the patient. The presence of a cervical fibroid in this patient was assessed and confirmed through vaginal and ultrasound examination, respectively. The use of other imaging methods (e.g., magnetic resonance imaging) for intraoperative mapping has been described in several reported cases. In the present case, considering the patient's surgical history, it may have been useful to have a comprehensive view of the adhesion. Another diagnostic method available is hysteroscopy, which may be useful for small-sized cervical fibroids [8]. However, for large-sized fibroids, as in the present case, it was not possible to use this modality due to the limitation of view. Notably, the patient did not wish to preserve her fertility. Based on this choice and the patient's age, we eventually performed hysterectomy. As reported by Nakayama et al., hysterectomy through the laparoscopic approach is applicable in this type of patients [9]. For this case, laparotomy was selected based on the preference of the surgeon. The histopathological results revealed the presence of condensed smooth muscle fibers confined within a pseudocapsule, which confirmed the diagnosis of the cervical fibroid.

In the previous surgery, a Pfannenstiel incision was performed. The patient was diagnosed with concurrent endometriosis at another hospital. Treating physicians should be aware of the possibility of severe adhesion in the internal genitalia. The Pfannenstiel incision is inferior to medial incision in terms of exposure. Therefore, its use is not recommended under certain conditions, and alternative access options are required to perform adhesiolysis [10]. The most challenging part is the location of cervical fibroids, which are close to other important structures (i.e., bladder at the anterior, rectum at the posterior, and ureters at the lateral side). The precise location of fibroids should be well defined, considering their importance in predicting anatomical alterations of the surrounding structures. There may be distortion of the normal anatomy of uterine vessels, pulling of the bladder, and distortion of the ureter. Enucleation of fibroids, followed by hysterectomy, may be a favorable treatment option to minimize injuries. However, this approach is linked to increased blood loss. Thus, this type of intervention is not recommended for patients with blood-borne diseases such as hepatitis C [11].

REFERENCES

[1] Stewart, E. A. (2013). Epidemiology, clinical manifestation, diagnosis, and natural history of uterine leiomyomas (fibroid). *Uptodate*.

[2] Hoffman, B., Schorge, J. and Schaffer, J. Pelvic Mass. (2012). In Williams Gynecology. *McGrawHill*, 2nd ed.

[3] Patel, P., Banker, M. and Munshi, S. (2011). Handling cervical myomas. *Journal of Gynecological Endoscopy and Surgery*, 2: 30 - 32.

[4] Vilos, G. A., Allaire, C., Laberge, P. Y. and Leyland, N. (2015). The management of uterine leiomyoma. *Journal of Obstetrics and Gynaecology Canada*, *37*: 157 - 178.

[5] Mendiratta, S., Dash, S., Mittal, R. and Dath, S. (2017). Cervical fibroid: an uncommon presentation. *International Journal of Reproduction, Contraception, Obstetrics and Gynecology*, *6*.

[6] Khanam, S. A., Rashid, F. and Chowdhury, S. (2016). An unusually big cervical fibroid polyp: A case report. *Chattagram Maa-O-Shishu Hospital Medical College Journal*, *15*: 65 – 67.

[7] Booher, Morgan. Myomectomy of a large cervical fibroid in a patient desiring future fertility. *OBG Management*, *30*: 20 – 22.

[8] Lasmar, B. P., Lasmar, R. B. and Pillar, C. (2013). Office hysteroscopic cervical myomectomy. *Gynecological Surgery*, *10*: 219.

[9] Nakayama, K., Tsukao, M., Ishikawa, M., Ishibashi, T., Nakamura, K., Sanuki, K., Yamashita, H., Ono, R., Minamoto, T. and Kyo, S. (2017). Total laparoscopic hysterectomy for large uterine cervical myoma. *Molecular and Clınıcal Oncology*, *6*: 655 - 660.

[10] Burke, J. J. and Gallup, D. G. (2008). Incision of gynecological surgery. In Rock, J. A., Jones, H. W., editors. *TeLinde's Operative Gynecology*. 10th ed. Philadelphia: Lippincott Williams and Wilkins

[11] El-Agwany, A. S. and Swelam, M. S. (2014). Unusual giant central cervical leiomyoma: a description of two cases. *Archives of Perinatal Medicine*, *20*: 113 - 115.

In: Obstetric and Gynecology Case Report
Editor: Dwiana Ocviyanti
ISBN: 978-1-53616-711-5

Chapter 21

RARE CASE OF INCISIONAL SITE ABDOMINAL WALL METASTASIS FROM UTERINE CERVICAL CANCER RECURRENCE DISEASE: A CASE REPORT AND LITERATURE REVIEW

Tofan Widya Utami**, Kade Yudi Saspriyana, Alvin Bramantyo and Gatot Purwoto

Department of Obstetric and Gynecology, Faculty of Medicine, Universitas Indonesia, Dr. Cipto Mangunkusumo Hospital, Jakarta, Indonesia

ABSTRACT

Cervical cancer most commonly recurs in the parametrium, pelvic lymph nodes, and vagina. The incidence of incisional skin metastasis from

* Corresponding Author's E-mail: tofanwidya@yahoo.com.

cervical cancer is extremely rare and usually results in a poor prognosis. A 54-year-old female patient was referred with an abdominal mass after definitive treatment for cervical cancer. Fourteen months before admission, she underwent radical hysterectomy with bilateral salpingo-oophorectomy and pelvic lymphadenectomy. Her abdominal examination at presentation revealed a 2 cm diameter mobile mass with solid consistency. Her fine needle aspiration biopsy results were positive for metastatic carcinoma. The patient was then given chemotherapy, at the end of which the mass still existed. We then performed wide excision of the mass followed by re-radiation therapy. Metastasis of the incisional site after definitive therapy for cervical cancer is an extremely rare occurrence in the follow-up of tumor patients and represents a challenge for the interdisciplinary team. Factors that affect the recurrence time, optimal management, and prognosis in these cases must be further studied.

Keywords: incisional site metastasis, recurrence disease, cervical cancer

Introduction

Cervical cancer is the second most commonly diagnosed type and the third leading cause of cancer death among women in developing countries [1]. Cervical cancer mainly spreads through a direct lymphatics route. The parametrium, pelvic lymph nodes, and vagina are among the most common sites of cervical cancer recurrence [2]. Incisional site recurrences are extremely rare, with incidences ranging from 0.1% to 1.3% [3]. This finding usually constitutes a poor prognosis [4]. Here we report a rare case of recurrent cervical cancer in an incisional site.

Case Presentation

This manuscript was approved by the Ethics Committees of Cipto Mangunkusumo National Referral Hospital, and the participant provided written informed consent. The patient was a 54-year-old woman who was referred to the hospital with an abdominal mass after receiving definitive treatment for cervical cancer. The mass was first detected in October 2016.

There was no associated vaginal bleeding and micturition or defecation problems. Her vital signs were normal. The patient was conscious, and no abnormalities were revealed during the heart and lung auscultation. Her abdominal examination revealed a 2 cm diameter mobile mass with a solid consistency. The mass was located on the right lateral site of the previous low transverse incision. Her gynecological examination revealed a normal vaginal wall, stump, and rectal mucosa with no pelvic mass detected.

The patient was first diagnosed with cervical cancer stage IIA2 in August 2015. She then underwent radical hysterectomy with bilateral salpingo-oophorectomy and pelvic lymphadenectomy in a private hospital. Post-operative pathologic findings displayed squamous cell (non-keratinized) carcinoma of the cervix with positive pelvic lymph node involvement. External radiation was then performed 25 times between April and May of 2016 in Gatot Subroto Army Hospital in Jakarta. During her follow-up at Fatmawati General Hospital in Jakarta in October 2016, a palpable mobile mass of 1 cm diameter was found on the incisional site. Fine needle aspiration biopsy was then performed with a positive result for metastatic carcinoma. A six-series chemotherapy regime of paclitaxel-cisplatin was administered between December 2016 and May 2017 in Fatmawati General Hospital, Jakarta. However, at the end of chemotherapy, the mass remained. Then, she was referred to the Cipto Mangunkusumo National Referral Hospital. In May 2018, we performed resection of the incisional scar along with extirpation of the right superficial inguinal lymph nodes. The specimens were then sent to the pathology department. The results displayed free margins of the tumor mass and positive metastatic disease on all lymph nodes with positive lymph vascular invasion. The patient was then scheduled for adjuvant re-radiation therapy in the Radiotherapy Department with 25 series of external radiation.

The patient finished external radiation in September 2018, with minimal complaints. Her performance status was good. A physical examination revealed no palpable mass on the abdominal incision and good wound healing.

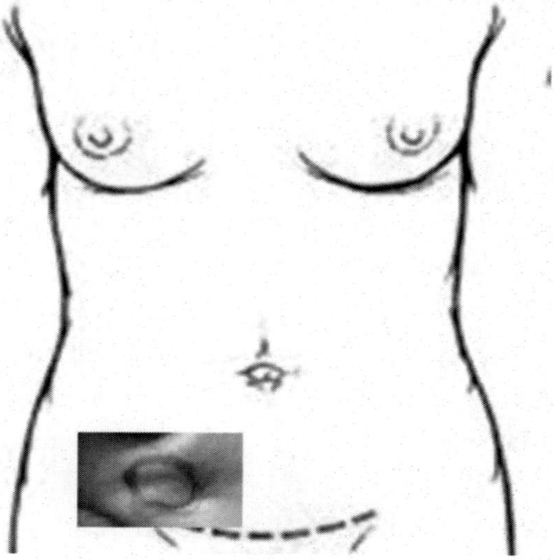

Figure 1. Schematic location of recurrent cervical cancer in the abdominal incision.

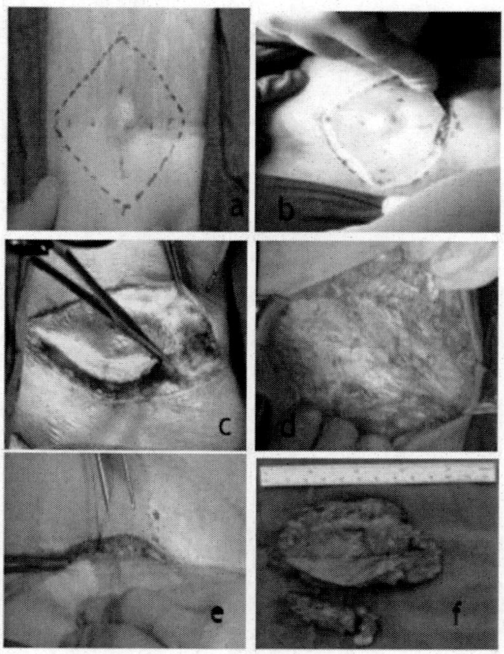

Figure 2. a. Preconstruction of surgery; b. beginning of the procedure; c. wide excision of the mass; d. after the mass was removed; e. after the procedure; f. the specimen.

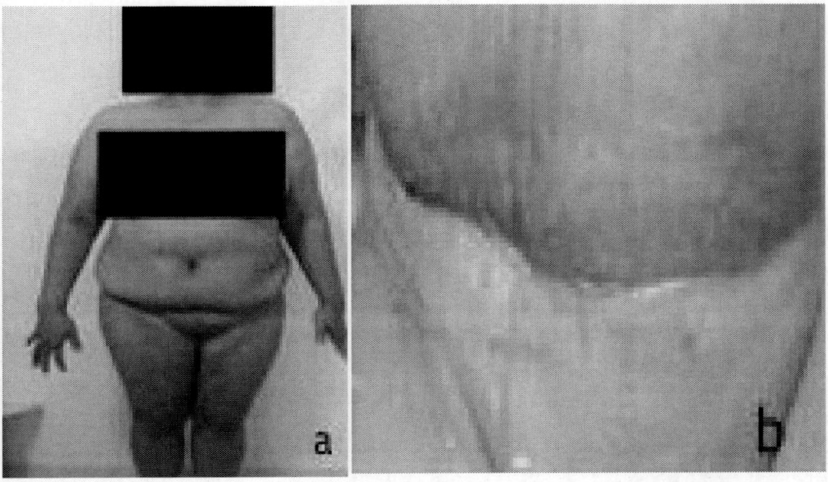

Figure 3. a. General performance after re-radiation; b. abdominal condition after re-radiation.

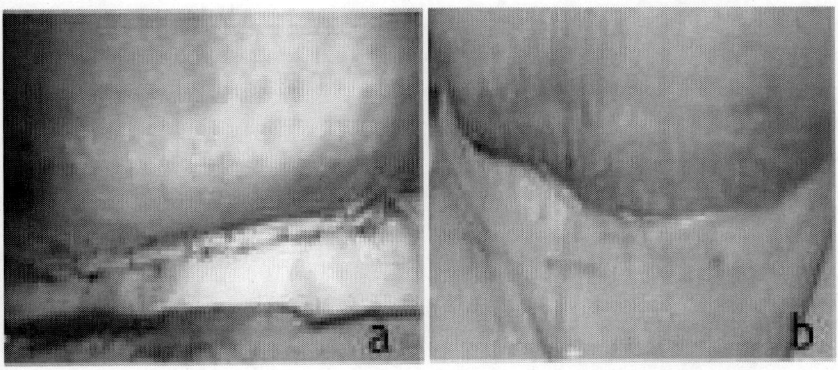

Figure 4. a. Abdominal condition after wide excision; b. abdominal condition after re-radiation.

DISCUSSION

Skin metastasis from cervical cancer is not a common manifestation and has an incidence rate of 5% or less [2]. The most common sites of skin lesions are the incisional site, vulva, and anterior chest wall [4]. Recurrence in the abdominal incisional site has been reported in cancers of the colon, gall bladder, kidney, and urinary bladder. However, cervical carcinoma rarely leads to such recurrence [5]. Aside from the laparotomy scar, cervical cancer recurrences have also been reported to develop on the laparoscopic port site, even for an unrelated laparoscopic surgery [6]. Recurrences of scar seem to be part of extensive metastatic [3]. Macroscopically, three common patterns (nodules, plaques, and inflammatory telangiectatic lesions) of skin metastasis have been observed [7]. Imachi et al., reported a mean interval between the diagnosis of cervical cancer and skin metastasis of 16.9 months [4]. Comparably, a recent case-control study showed that the mean time between surgery and the development of scar recurrence was 16 months [3]. Similar to the available literature, our patient developed the incisional site nodule 14 months after surgery. Adenocarcinomas compare to squamous cell carcinoma were found more commonly in skin metastatic. The incidence of skin metastasis from cervical cancer was 0.9% for cervical squamous cell carcinoma and 5.8% for cervical adenocarcinoma [4]. However, a recent case-control study reported that 9 out of 11 cervical cancer patients with scar recurrence displayed the squamous cell type [3].

Lavazzo et al., [8] clarified in their literature review that 1.5-45 months was range of recurrence (median 14 months). Wide excision was performed in 30/37 cases in which information regarding the treatment option was available, whereas 11/37 and 13/37 cases underwent radiotherapy and chemotherapy, respectively. The exact mechanism of how incisional site recurrence of cervical cancer develops is not yet fully understood. The possible mechanisms include iatrogenic tumor seeding at the time of surgery and circulating tumor cells trapped in the microcirculation of the wound. This is further aggravated by the inflammatory oncotaxis process that creates a favorable environment for the implantation and growth of tumor cells [3]. FIGO stage, involvement of the parametrium, positive resection margins, and a tumor diameter greater than 4 cm are factors that associated with a greater risk of disease recurrence [3].

There were four groups of potential risk factors of metastases: the first group relative to local immunoreactions, wound hypoxia, acidosis leading to angiogenesis and hematogenous spread around the navel. The second group includes characteristic of the disease (advanced disease, adenocarcinoma cell type, peritoneal carcinomatosis, and lymph node disease). There is a six-fold increased skin metastasis risk for stage IV disease compared with stage I disease. The seed and soil theory notes that cells can spread throughout the body via the blood or lymph vessels. Small number cell develop metastases depending on the tissue microenvironment and tumor type. The third group include to the surgical technique (mechanical port irrigation, no use of endobags, trocar size direct implantation by instruments or gloves). The last group includes factors of the laparoscopic environment (pneumoperitoneum condition and particularly the use of carbon dioxide) [8].

Currently, there are no guidelines for the treatment of incisional site cancer recurrence because of the limited number of cases reported. Treatment is mainly palliative and includes chemotherapy, radiotherapy, or wide surgical excision [8]. In our case, the patient was given re-radiation therapy after wide surgical excision of the recurrent tumor. However, patients who have undergone several operations or adjuvant therapies prior may have a worse physical condition that may affect the prognosis. Furthermore, patients who have had radiation therapy may go on to develop substantial wound healing deficits and necrosis, which may preclude sufficient local tissue being available for coverage; thus, the patient might require tissue transplantation from other sites [9].

The immune status of the host was also as one of the factors associated with the viability of the implanted tumor cells. The probability of occult tumor cells being present close to the local surgical wound created during the process of tumor resection higher than the probability of their presence in remote wounds, if the migration of tumor cells detached from the primary neoplasm within the developmentally defined morphogenetic unit [10]. Recurrences after tumor resection with microscopically free margins occur locally at the site of surgical resection in up to 50% of patients, whereas only 1-2% recurrences in the distant surgical scar. Neoplastic cells receive various stimuli and experience conditions favoring the formation of tumor relapse after exposed to the wound environment [11]. The current principles of surgical oncology must be revisited. A radical tumor operation must remove not only the macroscopic and microscopic tumor but also a maximum of the microscopically occult local cancer while causing minimal tissue trauma [11]. Prognosis in scar recurrent cervical cancer is poor because of the extensive disease. Ramirez et al., reported that 67% of patients died of the disease within a median follow-up period of 12 months [12]. However, there was no concurrent metastasis in our case. Therefore, our patient's survival may be better than that of other patients.

CONCLUSION

Metastasis of the incisional site is a rare occurrence in the follow-up of tumor patients and represents a challenge for the interdisciplinary team. Here we report successful treatment of abdominal incisional site recurrence of cervical cancer. Factors affecting the recurrence time, optimal management, and prognosis, in this case, must be further studied.

Using an excellent surgical technique during radical hysterectomy, particularly regarding instrument and tissue handling, is important to prevent the possibility of iatrogenic tumor seeding at time of surgery and circulating tumor cells trapped in the microcirculation of the wound. These strategies could reduce the incidence of incisional site metastasis.

FUNDING

The authors received no specific grant from any funding agency in the public, commercial, or not-for-profit sectors.

CONFLICT OF INTEREST

The authors declare no conflicts of interest in preparing this article.

REFERENCES

[1] Marth C, Landoni F, Mahner S, McCormack M, Gonzalez-Martin A, Colombo N. (2017). Cervical cancer: ESMO Clinical Practice Guidelines for diagnosis, treatment and follow-up. *Ann. Oncol. Off. J. Eur. Soc. Med. Oncol,* 28(iv) : 72–83.

[2] Srivastava K, Singh S, Srivastava M, Srivastava AN. (2005). Incisional skin metastasis of a squamous cell cervical carcinoma 3.5 years after radical treatment-A case report. *Int. J. Gynecol. Cancer*, 15:1183–6.

[3] Van Den Tillaart SAHM, Schoneveld A, Peters IT, Trimbos JBM, Van Hylckama Vlieg A, Fleuren GJ, et al. (2010). Abdominal scar recurrences of cervical cancer: incidence and characteristics: a case-control study. *Int. J. Gynecol. Cancer*, 20:1031–40.

[4] Imachi M, Tsukamoto N, Kinoshita S, Nakano H. (1993). Skin metastasis from carcinoma of the uterine cervix. *Gynecol. Oncol,* 48: 349–54.

[5] Sharma DN, Chawla S, Chander S, Gairola M, Thulkar S, Singh MK. (2000). Cervical carcinoma recurring in an abdominal wall incision. *Clin. Oncol,* 12:354–6.

[6] Kharod S, Yeung A, Fredenburg K, Greenwalt J. (2015). Cervical cancer with a rare umbilical metastases in prior surgical site. *Int. J. Surg. Case Rep,* 17: 8–11.

[7] Malfetano JH. (1986). Skin metastases from cervical cancer: a fatal event. *Gynecol. Oncol,* 24:177–82.

[8] Iavazzo C, Madhuri K, Tailor a, Butler-Manuel S. (2012). Incisional site metastasis in a patient with cervical carcinoma: a case report and review of the literature. *Case Rep. Obstet. Gynecol,* 593732. Available from: http://www.pubmedcentral.nih. gov/articlerender.fcgi?artid= 3513724&tool=p mcentrez&rendertype= abstract.

[9] Boos AM, Beckmann MW, Horch RE, Beier JP. (2014). Interdisciplinary treatment for cutaneous abdominal wall metastasis from cervical cancer with resection and reconstruction of the

abdominal wall using free latissimus dorsi muscle flap: a case report. *Geburtshilfe Frauenheilkd,* 74: 574–8.

[10] Arora RS, Dave KS, Chauhan A, Bhansali RP, Patel J. (2013). Abdominal scar recurrence of squamous cell carcinoma of cervix following simple hysterectomy. *J. Obstet. Gynecol. India*, 64:129–31.

[11] Höckel M, Dornhöfer N. (2005). The hydra phenomenon of cancer: Why tumors recur locally after microscopically complete resection. *Cancer Res,* 65:2997–3002.

[12] Ramirez PT, Frumovitz M, Wolf JK, Levenback C. (2004). Laparoscopic port-site metastases in patients with gynecological malignancies. *Int. J. Gynecol. Cancer*, 14: 1070–7.

In: Obstetric and Gynecology Case Report ISBN: 978-1-53616-711-5
Editor: Dwiana Ocviyanti

Chapter 22

HOW TO DIAGNOSE AND MANAGE MALIGNANT MELANOMA OF THE VAGINA, AN AGGRESSIVE MELANOMA: AN EVIDENCE-BASED CASE REPORT AND REVIEW

Tofan Widya Utami*[*], Herdhana Suwartono, Yohanes Handoko and Laila Nuranna
Department of Obstetric and Gynecology, Faculty of Medicine, Universitas Indonesia, Dr. Cipto Mangunkusumo Hospital, Jakarta, Indonesia

ABSTRACT

To determine the diagnostic modality and therapeutic management of malignant vaginal melanomas.

[*] Corresponding Author's E-mail: tofanwidya@yahoo.com.

Evidence-based case report and review, with literature from the PubMed and Cochrane databases. We identified 36 studies, of which seven could be evaluated. One serial case report concluded that melanoma should be diagnosed histopathologically and treated with local resection as the primary treatment, followed by chemotherapy as an adjuvant therapy; a median survival of 419 days post-therapy was reported.

One systematic review did not identify significant differences in survival time after radical excision compared with wide local excision (WLE) (median 33 vs. 19 months, P = 0.065). Four studies concluded that wide excisions with thorough removal of the macroscopic tumor and negative-free margins have better survival rates than treatment with primary radiotherapy, and in advanced-stage melanoma cases, palliative chemotherapy is preferred. In any patient with suspected vaginal melanoma, diagnosis should be established by histopathological examination, and staging should be determined based on pelvic examination and radiology work-up.

All patients with vaginal cancer should be referred to and treated by a multidisciplinary gynecological oncology team, with WLE as the recommended treatment and chemotherapy and radiation for unresectable cases.

Palliative chemoradiation should be considered for advanced-stage disease.

Keywords: vaginal cancer, malignant melanoma of the vagina, diagnosis, treatment

INTRODUCTION

Vaginal cancer constitutes < 2% of all gynecological cancers. Aggressive melanomais relatively rare, although it accounted for more than 13,200 cases in 2002; the incidence rate does not exceed 0.8 per 100,000 women worldwide.

The most frequent type of vaginal cancer is squamous cell carcinoma (~80%) [1] ollowed by adenocarcinoma (14%) (which occurs more commonly in younger women and children); the remaining 6% of cases are clear cell carcinoma, verrucous carcinoma, melanoma, and sarcoma [2].

Vaginal melanoma has not been studied as thoroughly before as necessary. Therefore, this study assessed the diagnostic and management procedures that can be performed to properly treat these patients.

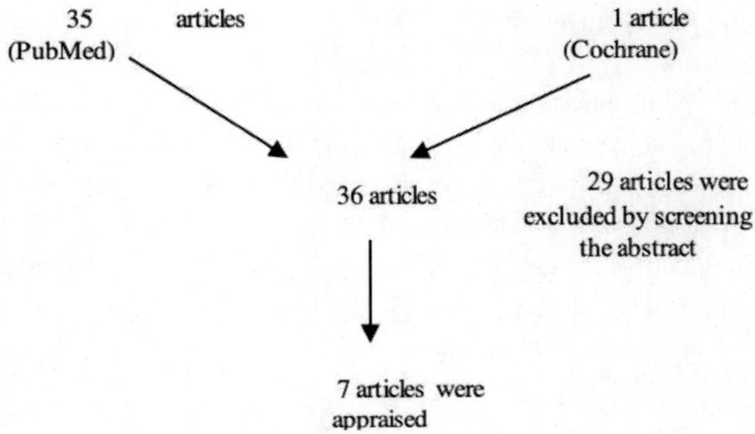

Figure 1. Literature search flowchart.

CASE REPORT

From 2017 to 2018, three cases of malignant vaginal melanoma were diagnosed at Cipto Mangunkusumo General Hospital (RSCM), which is a National Referral Hospital in Jakarta, Indonesia. Two of the cases continued treatment at the hospital, and one did not return after the initial visit. Of the two cases receiving treatment, one was a 59-year-old patient with melanoma of the vagina proven histopathologically by mass biopsy; the patient underwent neoadjuvant treatment with carboplatin and paclitaxel after previously receiving wide local excision (WLE). The other was a 38-year-old patient with vaginal melanoma diagnosed by histopathology and immunohistochemistry; she underwent external radiation. Currently, both patients have received their respective treatments and are being routinely assessed as scheduled.

METHODS

From the background information provided above, the research question of this study is the following: what isthe best diagnostic modality and therapeutic management for patients with malignant vulvar and vaginal melanoma?

To answer this question, we performed a search in the PubMed database for literature published in the last five years using four keywords with the MESH method: ("Malignant"[Mesh]) AND "Melanoma"[Mesh]) AND "Vagina"[Mesh]) AND "Diagnosis"[Mesh]). We also searched the Cochrane database using the MeSH descriptor as follows: [Malignant Melanoma] explode all trees AND MeSH descriptor: [Vagina] explode all trees AND MeSH descriptor: [Diagnostic].

RESULTS

Our literature search identified five studies that matched our research question and selection criteria. The first study wasa case series by Tasaka et al. [3], who reported on five patients with vaginal melanoma who were treated at the Department of Gynecology of Osaka City University Hospital between October 2000 and April 2014. On the basis of the validity and applicability of Tasaka et al. Study, we found that the focused research questions were clearly delineated, which was to evaluate the treatment of vaginal melanoma.

The rarity of vaginal melanoma cases prompts the use of case series, which is the method of this current study. The selection criteria of this study are the same as those for this case report evaluation: vaginal melanoma patients. In the study of Tasaka et al., the endpoints were the patients' outcome of survival or death from the disease, the disease-free survival (DFS) measured in days, and the overall survival (OS) measured in days.

All patients underwent local resection followed by adjuvant chemotherapy, ranging from DAVFeronto interferon beta. All patients displayed disease recurrence, with various sites of recurrence such as the uterus and cervix, pelvic lymph nodes, liver, brain, and lung. Only one patient evaluated survived until the study. The median OS was 419 days, and the median DFS was 177 days.

Table 1. Validity and applicability of the studies included in the analysis (1)

Study	Study Type	Focused Research Question	Selection Criteria	Primary Outcome
Tasaka et al., 2017 [3]	Research article	Yes	Yes	Analyzed five patients with vaginal melanoma
Rouzbahman et al., 2015 [4]	Research article	Yes	Yes	Analyzed five patients with vaginal melanoma
Aulmann et al., 2015 [5]	Research article	Yes	Yes	Established biological properties and evaluated potential therapeutic targets in vulvar and vaginal melanomas
Rapi et al., 2016 [10]	Case report and systematic literature review	Yes	Yes	Stages treated by surgery, radiotherapy, chemotherapy, or radiochemotherapy
Skovsted et al., 2017 [11]	Retrospective cohort study	Yes	Yes	Average time diagnosis, median survival, five-year survival rate
Todo et al., 2016 [6]	Systematic review	Yes	Yes	Overall survival, radicality of the initial surgery (RAINS) score
Kalampokus et al., 2017 [7]	Case report	Yes	Yes	Efficient treatment

The second study was performed by Rouzbahman et al. [4] and evaluated the molecular characteristics of malignant vaginal melanoma, specifically the frequency of the BRAF, C-KIT, and NRAS mutations. This study was a retrospective review of vulvar (n = 15) and vaginal (n = 5) melanoma cases obtained from the pathology database of the University Health Network (Toronto General Hospital, Princess Margaret Cancer Centre, and Toronto Western Hospital) of Canada between 2002 and 2013. These cases had undergone clinical and histological evaluation, continuing with genotyping studies on cases with cancer tissues available. The authors found that of the five vaginal cases, only a specific TP53 gene mutation was present (in four cases); the results for the fifth case were inconclusive. Statistical correlation analysis did not find any significant relationships between the mutation status and the patients'clinical or histological findings such as depth of invasion, ulceration, stage at presentation, or lymph node metastasis [4].

The findings by Rouzbahman et al. stood out in comparison to another study conducted by Aulmann et al. [5], who performed a case series of 65 cases from 1985 to 2010 at three centers: Heidelberg University Hospital and Tuebingen University Hospital (both in Germany) and the University of British Columbia Hospital (in Vancouver, Canada). This study evaluated the clinical, pathological, and molecular features of vulvar (n = 50) and vaginal (n = 15) melanoma cases.

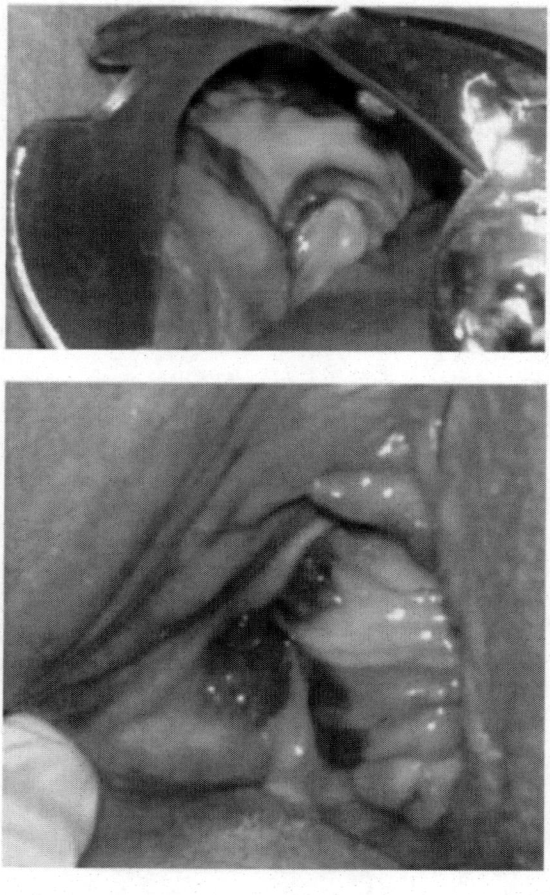

Figure 2. Suspected vaginal cancer that begins with malignant melanoma.

Tumor type, presence of ulceration, cellularity, pigmentation, tumor depth, lymph node status, molecular findings, presence of KIT gene immunohistochemistry (IHC) study, follow-up time, and status of these cases were studied. Of the 15 vaginal melanoma cases, NRAS G12V and Q61H amplification were identified in two cases and KIT amplification was identified in two cases.

The NRAS G12V and KIT genes were amplified simultaneously in one case. Despite these findings, the authors reported that none of the molecular features, such as KIT or NRAS, were associated with patient survival based on follow-up time and status, and only one patient was alive by the time of the study. Greater tumor depth (> 10mm) and the presence of lymph node metastases were significantly associated with poorer patient outcome, which was classified by survival status and length of survival time.

An evidence-based case report similar to our study was conducted by Todo et al. [5] who assessed the radicality of the initial surgery (RAINS) score and the survival outcomes of 147 malignant vaginal melanoma patients from 1975 to 2014 in the MEDLINE and EMBASE published reports.

This study evaluated validity and applicability based on the clinical question of determining the negative consequences of radical surgery, which was assessed from the association between a higher RAINS score (> 7) and the patients' OS time. This study found that patients with a higher RAINS score had a significantly longer survival time than those with a RAINS score ofless than 7 (median survival time 41 vs. 19 months, P = 0.037). Furthermore, the group of patients with a RAINS score of at least 7 included significantly more patients with advanced-stage disease than the group of patients with a RAINS score of 6 or less (38 vs. 16%, P = 0.023). However, this systematic review showed that there was no significant difference in OS between patients with a RAINS score of 6 or higher and those with a score of 5 or less (median survival time, 33 vs. 19 months; log-rank test, P = 0.065) [6].

Table 2. Validity of the studies included in the analysis (2)

Study	Overall Results (treatment preference)	OR	95% CI
Tasaka et al., 2017 [3]	Local resection, thermal injection with interferon beta (n=3), dacarbazine, nimustine, vin cristine, and interferon beta (n=1)	–	–
Rouzbahman et al., 2015 [4]	BRAF mutations are infrequent, whereas C-KIT and NRAS mutations are observed with a higher frequency in vulvar melanomas than in melanomas of other sites	Statistically not significant	–
Aulmann et al., 2015 [5]	KIT mutations were exclusively observed in vulvar melanomas (P=0.171)	–	–
Rapi et al., 2016 [10]	No evidence of disease, and the patient is still alive	–	–
Skovsted et al., 2017 [11]	Median diagnosed age was older, low five-year survival rate, poor prognosis	–	–
Todo et al., 2016 [6]	Overall survival with a RAINS score of at least 7 was significantly longer that that with a RAINS score of 6 or less (median survival time, 41 vs. 19 months: log-rank test, (P = 0.037). Asignificant difference in overall survival was not found between patients with a RAINS score of 6 or more or 5 or less	–	–
Kalampokus et al., 2017 [7]	Surgery	–	–

Treatment for this condition was described in a case report by Kalampokas et al. [7] on a 75-year-old Caucasian woman para 2, from Athens, Greece, who was subjected to WLE surgery with at least 1.5cm of free margins without any adjuvant therapy such as radiotherapy or chemotherapy. The patient underwent postoperative histological diagnosis confirmation by positive IHC staining for S-100 and MART-1, which was confirmed as primary malignant vaginal melanoma with clear surgical margins. The authors concluded that WLE seems to be the only efficient treatment according to the results from the patient's follow-up 12 months after the initial diagnosis and at three-month intervals after WLE. At those times, the clinical examination and CTscan of the chest, abdomen, and pelvis presented no signs of disease recurrence [7].

DISCUSSION

The five studies that we evaluated from1975 to 2014 included a total of 173 cases. The follow-up time of the studies ranged from 16 months to 39 years, with a mean study duration of 18.05 years. The overall results demonstrated that limited studies with high-level evidence have been performed, such as those based on randomized controlled trialsor meta-analyses. This finding is a result of the rarity of vaginal melanoma cases worldwide. For example, data from the Bishop et al. population-based analysis [8] conclude that vaginal cancer constitutes less than 2% of gynecological cancers, with the aggressive form of melanoma accounting for only approximately 13,200 cases. Because of the lack of cases that can be evaluated, all the studies that we identified were in the form of case reports or case series. However, these studies were still valuable in our estimations because of the thoroughness of the evaluations shown by the lengthy periods of follow-up, complete follow-up on the survival of patients, and the varieties of data that were presented, ranging from molecular and genetic studies to clinical evaluations of diagnosis and treatments. The studies mentioned in this analysis showed that conventional diagnostic methods such as histopathological examination, staging based on pelvic examination and radiology work-up (CTscan or MRI), and referral and treatment in a gynecological oncology center (GOC) by a multidisciplinary gynecological oncology team are still the preferred procedures for vaginal melanoma cases. From the molecular studies of Rouzbahman et al. [4] and Aulmann et al. [5], we can conclude that there are no satisfactory molecular and genetic markers that are significantly correlated with specific vaginal melanoma diagnostic indicators. According tothe European Society of Gynecology Oncology (ESGO) [9], the main diagnostic procedure is based on histopathological and pelvic examination, supplemented with radiology work-up.

The recommended treatment of WLE is still the primary treatment available, with definitive chemoradiation (with radiation dose escalation) as the treatment of choice in patients with unresectable disease. According to the ESGO guidelines on vaginal melanoma, adjuvant chemoradiation, which includes platinum-based chemotherapy such as carboplatin, cisplatin, or paclitaxel, can also be considered. One study by Kalampokas et al. [7] did not continue with adjuvant chemoradiation; however, this study had a very limited follow-up compared with the other studies presented, and thus we can conclude that adjuvant treatments are still valuable. Notably, the use of adjuvant treatments is based on the clinical judgments of the gynecologists themselves.

Table 3. Importance of the studies included in the analysis

Study	Study Design	Number of Subjects	Validity Appraisal	Intervention	Duration of Follow-up	Applicability
Tasaka et al., 2017 [3]	Prospective study	5	Yes	Local resection followed by adjuvant therapy	1 year	Yes
Rouzbahman et al., 2015 [4]	Prospective review	44	Yes	–	–	No
Aulmann et al., 2015 [5]	Descriptive	65	Yes	–	–	No
Rapi et al., 2016 [10]	Prospective	1	Yes	Surgery, vaginal brachytherapy 50 Gy	< 12 months	Yes
Skovsted et al., 2017 [11]	Retrospective	17	Yes	–	84 months	Yes
Todo et al., 2016 [6]	Retrospective	31 studies and 157 subjects	Yes	–	–	Yes
Kalampokus et al., 2017 [7]	Descriptive	1	Yes	Surgery	12 months	Yes

These findings correspond with a case series by Miner et al. [9] who demonstrated that women with primary vaginal melanoma who underwent surgery first had a better median survival compared with those in whom primary radiotherapy was performed when survival was calculated at 20 months. This finding indicates that WLE is still understandably considered the primary treatment for vaginal melanoma. The thorough removal of the macroscopic tumor and negative-free margins were found to be effective in guaranteeing local control and improving survival [9]. Kalampokas et al. also found that in advanced stages of vaginal melanoma or with deteriorating health conditions of the patients, palliative chemotherapy is preferred. Postoperative adjuvant therapy, such as IF-2b, radiotherapy, and chemotherapy, has been effective in preventing tumors from relapsing [7].

CONCLUSION

In any patient with suspected vaginal melanoma, diagnosis should be established by histopathological examination. Staging should be based on pelvic examination and radiology work-up (CTscan or MRI). All patients with suspected malignant vaginal melanoma should be referred to a GOC and treated by a multidisciplinary gynecological oncology team. Radical local excision is recommended. Definitive chemoradiation (with radiation dose escalation) is the treatment of choice in patients with unresectable disease. Moreover, for advanced-stage disease, the ESGO guidelines on vaginal melanoma recommend considering neoadjuvant chemoradiation, which includes platinum-based chemotherapy such as carboplatin, cisplatin, orpaclitaxel.

REFERENCES

[1] Creasman, W. T., Phillips, J. L., Menck, H. R. (1998). The National Cancer Data Base report on cancer of the vagina. *Cancer*, 83: 1033 - 1040.

[2] Piura, B. (2008). Management of primary melanoma of the female urogenital tract. *Lancet oncology,* 9: 973 - 981.

[3] Tasaka, R., Fukuda, T., Wada, T., Kawanishi, M., Imai, K., Kasai, M. et al. (2017). A retrospective clinical analysis of 5 cases of vaginal melanoma. *Molecular and clinical oncology*, 6: 373 - 376.

[4] Rouzbahman, M., Kamel-Reid, S., Al Habeeb, A., Butler, M., Dodge, J., Laframboise, S. et al. (2015). Malignant melanoma of vulva and vagina. *Journal of lower genital tract disease*, 19: 350 - 353.

[5] Aulmann, S., Sinn, H. P., Penzel, R., Gilks, C. B., Schott, S., Hassel, J. C. et al. (2014). Comparison of molecular abnormalities in vulvar and vaginal melanomas. *Modern pathology*, 27: 1386 - 1393.

[6] Todo, Y., Okamoto, K., Suzuki, Y., Minobe, S., Kato, H. (2016). Radicality of initial surgery for primary malignant melanoma of the vagina. *Melanoma research*, 26:173 - 180.

[7] Kalampokas, E., Kalampokas, T., Damaskos, C. (2017). Primary vaginal melanoma, a rare and aggressive entity. A case report and review of the literature. *In Vivo*, 31: 133 - 140.

[8] Bishop, K. D., Olszewski, A. J. (2014). Epidemiology and survival outcomes of ocular and mucosal melanomas: A population-based analysis. *International journal of cancer*, 134: 2961 - 2971.

[9] Miner, T. J., Delgado, R., Zeisler, J., Busam, K., Alektiar, K., Barakat, R. et al. (2004). Primary vaginal melanoma: A critical analysis of therapy. *Annals of surgical oncology*, 11: 34 - 39.

[10] Rapi, V., Dogan, A., Schultheis, B., Hartmann, F., Rezniczek, G. A., Tempfer, C. B. (2017). Melanoma of the vagina: Case report and systematic review of the literature. *Anticancer Research*, 37: 6911 - 6920.

[11] Skovsted, S., Nielsen, K., Blaakær, J. (2017). Melanomas of the vulva and vagina. *Danish medical journal*: 64.

In: Obstetric and Gynecology Case Report ISBN: 978-1-53616-711-5
Editor: Dwiana Ocviyanti

Chapter 23

ACQUIRED LABIAL FUSION MIMICKING CONGENITAL UROGENITAL SINUS ANOMALY: A CASE REPORT

Fernandi Moegni*

Department of Obstetric and Gynecology, Faculty of Medicine, Universitas Indonesia, Dr. Cipto Mangunkusumo Hospital, Jakarta, Indonesia

ABSTRACT

The diagnosis of labial fusion is sometimes difficult. Total closure of the vaginal opening because of dense adhesion can be misdiagnosed as congenital urogenital sinus or Mullerian anomaly. An incorrect diagnosis may result in the patient receiving wrong information and an inappropriate treatment. Here we report a case of labial fusion in a 34-year-old woman. She was referred with an initial diagnosis of congenital urogenital sinus anomaly (low vaginal septum). On history taking, she mentioned frequent vulvar erosion during bicycle riding in her adolescence. On physical

* Corresponding Author's E-mail: fernandi71@ui.ac.id.

examination, total labial fusion was noted, with only a pinpoint hole. Additionally, on ultrasound, all structures at the vulvo-vaginal area could be distinguished. Thus, a final diagnosis of labial fusion was made. She underwent appropriate surgery without any complications. In such cases, careful history taking, physical examination, and transrectal ultrasound imaging can help make an accurate diagnosis of labial fusion and help patient achieve appropriate management to relieve all the symptoms.

Keywords: labial fusion, congenital urogenital sinus, Mullerian anomaly

INTRODUCTION

Labial fusion is a condition characterized by partial or complete adherence of the labia minora in prepubertal girls [1]. This condition can also occur in postmenopausal women and even in women of reproductive age [2, 3]. Many symptoms could arise because of these event such as micturition problems like voiding difficulty until urinary incontinence and also urinary retention [4, 5]. Other problem that was also reported is related with sexual dysfunction. [3].

The other problem happen with this event is the issue of how to determine the correct diagnosis of this kind of case. It is not rare and quite common that many health providers even specialist doctors have difficulty to determine the right diagnosis of this case because of the small number of case. This rare incident make it is little known or unnoticed by most of the doctors or parents because they even have not had such experience to recognize this genital appearance [6].

We report an interesting case of labial fusion in a woman of reproductive age. She was referred with an initial diagnosis of congenital urogenital sinus anomaly (low vaginal septum), but her final diagnosis was labial fusion.

CASE REPORT

A 34-year-old woman was referred to us with a diagnosis of congenital urogenital sinus anomaly. Her main complaint was inability to perform sexual intercourse since marriage (1.5 years ago). Another complaint was difficulty in micturition; she mentioned that passing of urine had become gradually obstructed, with reduced amount of urine passed each time. She had been examined by a doctor and was informed that she had congenital urogenital sinus anomaly. The diagnosis was made based on the finding of total closure of the vaginal opening, and she was planned to be referred to a urogynecologist for a complex reconstruction surgery because of this diagnosis, which made her anxious. At a tertiary-level health service, detailed menstrual history was taken, which was unremarkable. On being asked about having any chronic inflammation in the vulvar area, she mentioned frequent vulvar erosion during bicycle riding in her adolescence. She denied having frequent vaginal discharge or itching of the vulva at that time.

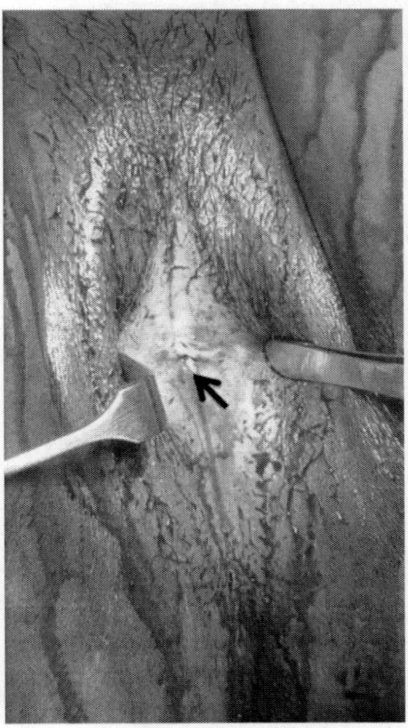

Figure 1. Image on physical examination. Total labial fusion is noted, with only a pinpoint hole (arrow).

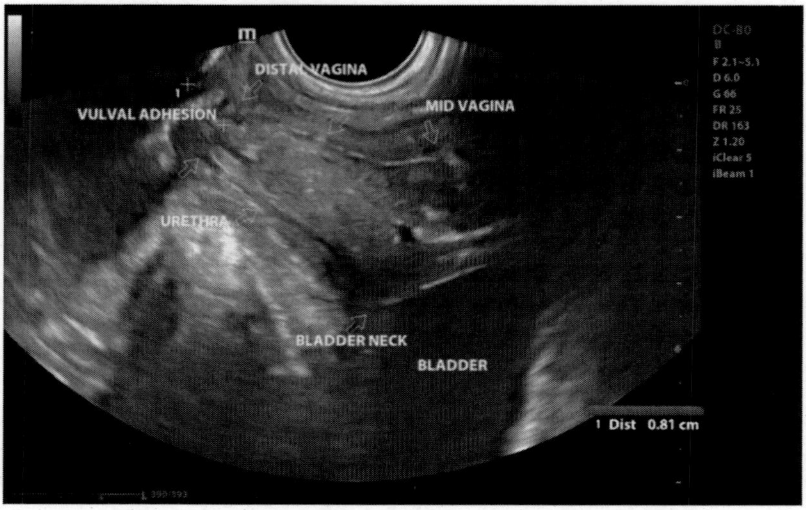

Figure 2. Transrectal ultrasound imagingrevealed normal vaginal canal, bladder, bladder neck, and urethra. Vulvar adhesion was noted in the distal area (0.81 cm).

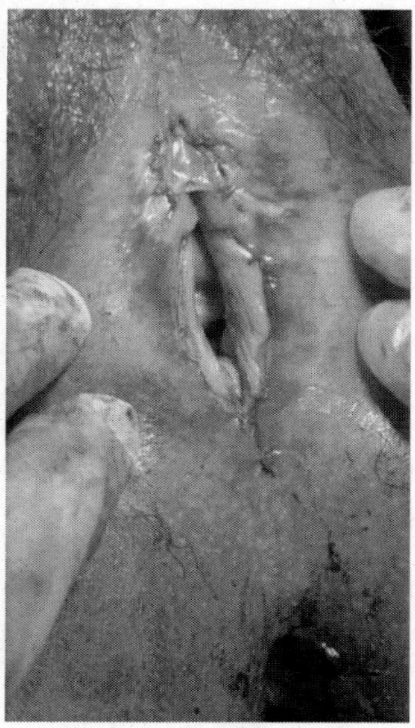

Figure 3. Vulva post labial fusion separation surgery.

On physical examination, the vaginal opening was found to be closed, with fusion of the labia minora and only a pinpoint hole (Figure 1). Rectal touche revealed a normal uterus and unremarkable findings at both adnexal areas.

Transrectal ultrasound revealed a normal vaginal canal and an unremarkable bladder and urethra. Adhesion was present at the labial area that could partially obstruct the flow of urine (Figure 2).

The patient under went surgery on day care basis. A labial incision was made, and the left and right labia minora were separated. The wound was sutured with polyglycolic acid suture no.3.0 (Figure 3).

DISCUSSION

Labial fusion usually occurs more frequently during childhood when estrogen is lacking. The mean age at occurrence is 2.5 years, with the condition occurring before the age of 6 years in 90% of the cases [7]. Around this age, the labia minora mucosa shows increased epithelialization but is not mature enough to achieve full thickness for the prevention of adhesion. Girls may have symptoms of micturition or vulvar pruritus [8] or may be asymptomatic [9].

Labial fusion also occurs frequently in women of postmenopausal age, again owing to the lack of estrogen [2]. Our case was that of a woman of reproductive age, which is similar to the case of labial fusion in a woman of reproductive age reported by Goldstein et al. [10]. Such cases are quite rare owing to the high estrogen levels present at reproductive age. Labial fusion around this time usually involves other causes, with the main cause being chronic inflammation possibly due to with chronic trauma [11]. In the present case, there was no vaginal discharge, nor infection, such as bacterial or fungal, was not found to be associated with chronic inflammation. However, our patient experienced chronic vulvar trauma associated with bicycle riding, which was believed to be the cause of labial fusion. The scar developed at the fusion location made it difficult to distinguish the condition from congenital urogenital sinus anomaly [6]. The initial diagnosis of congenital urogenital sinus anomaly was incorrect, and the patient became anxious after being informed about the complex surgery required based on this diagnosis. Eventually, the correct diagnosis of vulvar/labial adhesion was made with the help of ultrasound imaging that showed a normal vaginal structure. She underwent the appropriate surgery without any complications.

CONCLUSION

Labial fusion is a rare aquired case that can happen during childhood, reproductive age or postmenopausal age. The main etiologies of this condition are lack of estrogen hormone or chronic inflammation. It can make several problem in micturition such as voiding difficulty, urinary incontinence and urinary retention, and also problem in sexual intercourse. The other problem of this case is in determining the right diagnosis due to the similar appearance of it that can mimicking other diagnosis.

Acquired labial fusion is not common in women of reproductive age, and it might mimic congenital urogenital sinus anomaly, resulting in confusion regarding the correct diagnosis. In such cases, careful history taking, physical examination, and ultrasound imaging can help make an accurate diagnosis and help in appropriate management.

REFERENCES

[1] Ben-Ami, T., Boichis, H., Hertz, M., (1978). Fused labia. Clinical and radiological findings. *Pediatr. Radiol*, 7 : 33-35.

[2] Palla, L., De Angelis, B., Lucarini, L., Spallone, D., Palla, G., Cervelli, V., (2010). A case of labial fusion and urinary pseudo-incontinence in an elderly woman. A surgical treatment and a review. *Eur. Rev. Med. Pharmacol. Sci*, 14 : 491-493.

[3] Katageri Geetanjali, M., Pujari Linganand, L., Vishwanath, G., Doddamani, U., (2011). Apareunia due to labial adhesions: A rare postpartum complication. *J. Clin. Diagn. Res*, 5 : 1670-1671.

[4] Ong, N. C. S., Dwyer, P. L., (1999). Labial Fusion Causing Voiding Difficulty and Urinary Incontinence. *Aust. NZ J. Obstet. Gynecol,* 3: 391-393.

[5] Erdogdu, E., Demirel, C., Tahaoglu, A. E., Ozdemir, A., (2017). Labial fusion: A rare cause of urinary retention in reproductive age woman and review of literature. *Turk. J. Urol,* 43(1): 98-101.

[6] Knudtzon, S., Haugen, S. E., Myhre, A. K., (2017). Labial adhesion-diagnostics and treatment. [Article in English, Norwegian] *Tidsskr Nor Legeforen,* 137 : 31-35.

[7] Klein, V. R., Willman, S. P., Carr, B. R., (1989). Familial posterior labial fusion. *Obstet. Gynecol,* 73 : 500-502.

[8] Paek, S. C., Merritt, D. F., Mallory, S. B. (2001) Pruritus vulvae in prepubertal children. *J. Am. Acad. Dermatol,* 44: 795-802.

[9] Hamell-Teillac, D. (2004). Vulvo-Vaginal Disorders. In: Sultan C. (ed): Pediatric and Adolescent Gynecology. Evidence-Based Clinical Practice. *Endocr. Dev*. Basel, Karger, vol. 7: 39-56.

[10] Goldstein, A. I., Rajcher, W. J., (1972). Conglutination of the labia minora in the presence of normal endogenous estrogen levels: an exception to the rule. *Am. J. Obstet. Gynecol.* 113 : 845-846.

[11] Capraro, V. J., Greenberg, H., (1972). Adhesions ofthe labia minora. *Obstet. Gynecol.* 39 : 65-69.

In: Obstetric and Gynecology Case Report ISBN: 978-1-53616-711-5
Editor: Dwiana Ocviyanti

Chapter 24

EXTRAMAMMARY PAGET'S DISEASE

Tricia Dewi Anggraeni, Bella Aprilia, Gatot Purwoto, Sigit Purbadi and Laila Nuranna*

Department of Obstetric and Gynecology, Faculty of Medicine, Universitas Indonesia, Dr. Cipto Mangunkusumo Hospital, Jakarta, Indonesia

ABSTRACT

Extramammary Paget's disease is a rare malignant neoplasm that occurs in women. It arises from apocrine glan-bearing skin cells or manifestation of adjacent primary anal, rectal or bladder adenocarcinoma. A visible lesion is typically erythematous plaque occuring in external genitalia, which mimicks dermatology lesions. However due to its slow growth rate, it may cause delayed diagnosis then consequently worsen prognosis. Here, we present case of 46 year old woman with persistent reddish plaque in vulvar area for 1 year. The lesion was mimicking fungal infection that she received treatment from dermatologist. Biopsy result was extramammary Paget's disease. Patient received further biopsy lesion to determine the malignant area and then continue with a wide local excision

* Corresponding Author's E-mail: bellaraphael.md@gmail.com.

with keystone flap. Patient has routinely control to plastic surgeon clinic for further wound care.

Keywords: extramammary, Paget's disease, vulvar, excision

INTRODUCTION

Paget's disease of the vulva is a very rare malignant neoplasm that is most commonly observed in postmenopausal women [1]. It originates from apocrinegland-bearing skin cellsor as a manifestation of adjacent primary anal, rectal, or bladder adenocarcinoma [2]. Mammary Paget's disease involving the nipple and areola was first described by Sir James Paget in 1874 [3]. In 1889, Crocker reported the first case of extramammary Paget's disease affecting the scrotum and penis. Paget's disease of the vulva was first reported in France in 1901 by Dr. William Dubreuilth [4].

Nearly 90% of cases of Paget's disease are of mammary Paget's disease and the remaining are of extramammary PD (EMPD) [5]. The overall incidence of EMPD in Europe is 0.7 per 100,000 individuals per year, and the incidence is slightly higher in women than that in men. In Asia, EMPD most commonly occurs in men [6]. Approximately 17% – 30% of patients with EMPD have an underlying adenocarcinoma. The most common symptoms are pruritus, burning pain, lump, and occasionally a painful erosion [1]. A visible lesion, typically an erythematous plaque, is present in almost all patients. The labia majora are the most frequently involved sites, followed by the labia minora, clitoris, perineum, and the perineal area [4, 7].

In addition to a slow-growing presentation that sometimes causes a delay in diagnosis and consequently a worse prognosis, Paget's disease has a chronic and relapsing course. A definitive diagnosis is obtained using biopsy. The treatment of choice is surgery; however, the disease frequently extends beyond the visible lesion, and therefore, surgical margins are frequently positive [8]. Many patients undergo multiple surgical procedures, including wide local excision, simple vulvectomy, or radical vulvectomy [9]. Such treatments commonly require a challenging reconstruction.

However, to the best of our knowledge, there are currently no standard treatment guidelines as extramammary Paget's disease is uncommon.

CASE REPORT

A 46-year-old woman presented with an itchy, reddish area on the vulva that was persistent since approximately 1 year. She had been treated with antifungal and antiallergic agents; however, no improvement was observed and the affected area was increasing in size. The patient underwent a biopsy on October 26, 2016, and the pathology anatomy results showed a histologic pattern of extramammary Paget's disease.

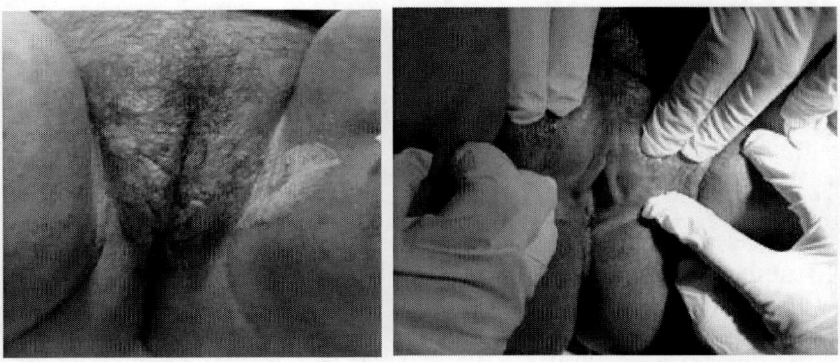

Figure 1. Clinical appearance of Paget's disease with normal urethral and vaginal mucosa.

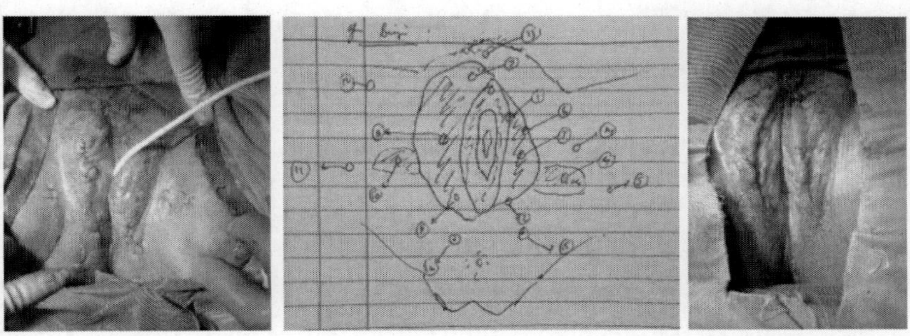

Figure 2.A. Eczematous lesion on the external genitalia. B. Biopsy mapping. C. Post-biopsy.

Physical examination revealed that the eczematous lesions had extended to the mons pubis, both the labias, and both thigh folds (Figure 1). Some areas showed prominent excoriations and lichenification. Some lesions progressed into sharply marginated plaque with distinct erythema. There was no involvement of the orificium urethrae externum, perineum, or anus. On March 16, 2017, the patient underwent skin lesion biopsy in the operating theater to determine the margin of excision (Figure 2 A–C).

Pathology Report

Histological examination demonstrated epithelial malignant tumor cells infiltrating the epidermis (Figure 3).

The local epidermis appeared to be ulcerative. The tumor cells were clustered in the local basal layer and filled the entire thickness of the epidermis. The tumor cells had large, pleomorphic, partially visible nucleoli. All surgical margins were negative.

Treatment Plan

Two months after biopsy mapping, the patient underwent wide local excision with keystone flap (Figure 4-6).

Six months after the surgery, the patient began to complain of difficulty in urinating. Physical examination revealed a unidentified vagina and vulva with labial fusion and small ostium. Subsequently, the patient underwent repair of the labial synechiae. The incision was performed around the ostium until the posterior vaginal wall could be seen. The urethra was identified and a urethral catheter was inserted. All scar lesions were excised and sent for pathological examination. The flap was then repaired and fixed to the labia majora, and a vaginal mold was inserted to prevent secondary synechiae. The patient continued to receive wound care from a plastic surgeon as well as the replacement of the vaginal mold every week.

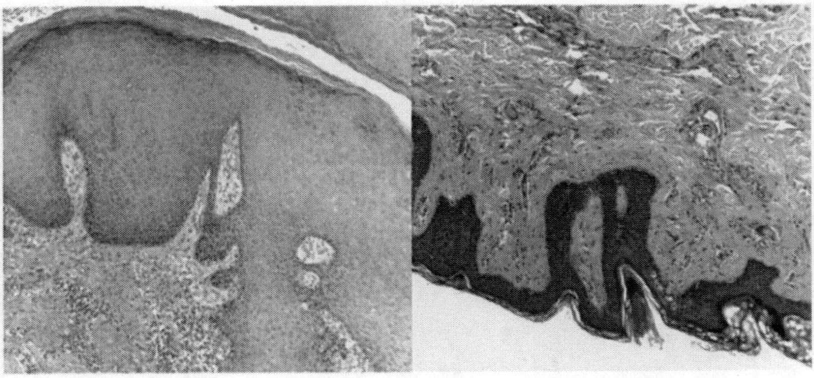

Figure 3. Histopathologic findings demonstrate squamous epithelial cells infiltrating the dermis with enlarged, eccentrically placed hyperchromatic nuclei and pale cytoplasm (magnification: left × 10, right × 100).

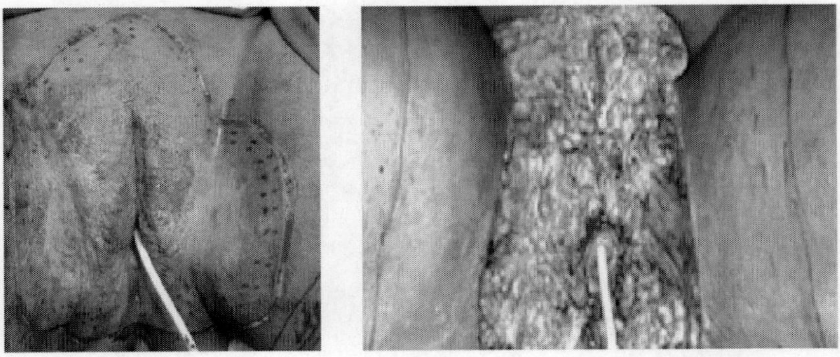

Figure 4. Left: design of incision. Right: view after wide local excision.

DISCUSSION

As Extramammary Paget's disease is very rare, there are no guidelines for its systematic workup and treatment. There are three theories regarding the origin of EMPD [1]. It is suggested to arise from the adnexal structures, such as the apocrine glands, multipotent stem cells in the epidermal basal layer, or infundibular stem cells of the hair follicles; from mammary like glands located in the interlabial sulci; or from the Toker cells, which are cells with a single round nucleus and pale cytoplasm that are usually found in the nipple and areola.

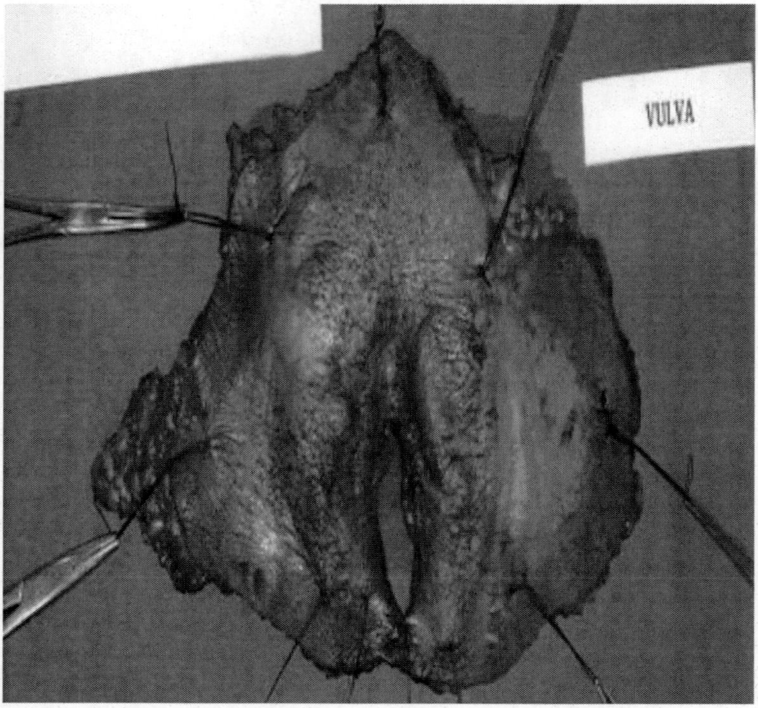

Figure 5. Gross macroscopic view of the excised tissue.

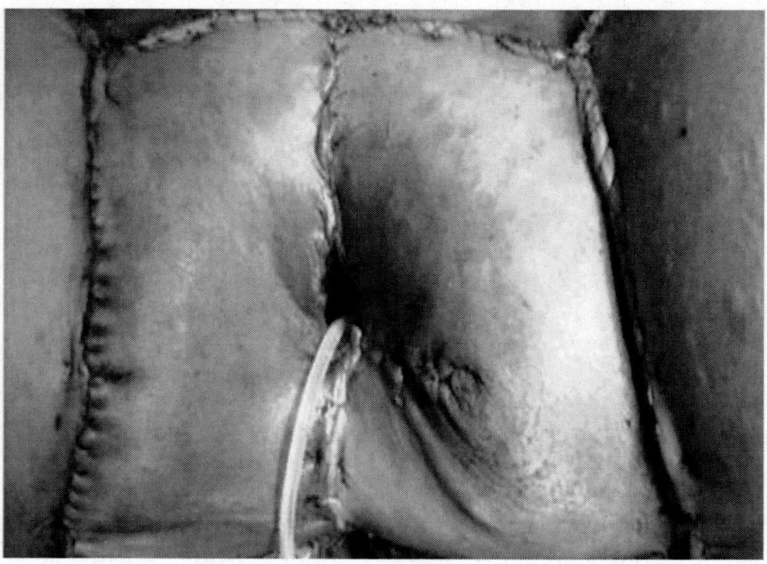

Figure 6. Defect closure with keystone flap.

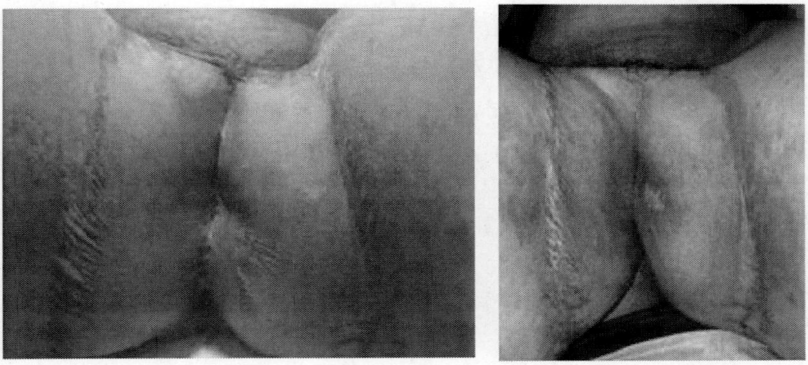

Figure 7. Clinical photographs 6 months after the surgery.

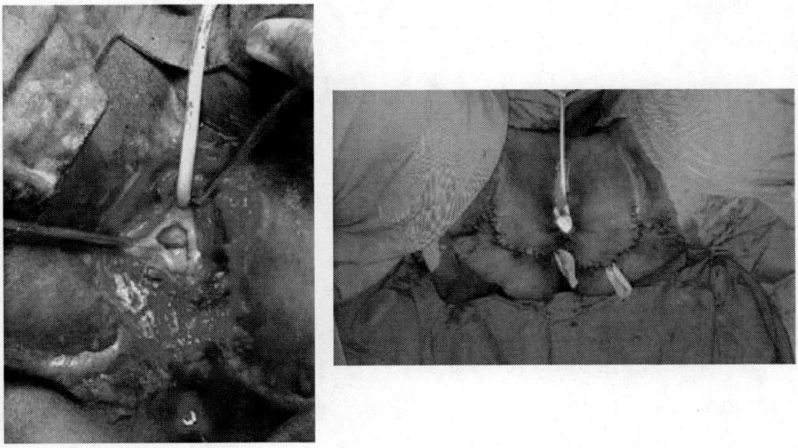

Figure 8. A. Repair of labial synechiae B. Postsurgical views.

Therefore, the vulva is the most common site of involvement. Classifications of the disease are based on the histological criteria proposed by Wilkinson et al. in 2002 [1, 10] (Table 1).

The workup for vulvar Paget's disease includes recording a history of vulvovaginal complaints and gastrointestinal and urologic symptoms as the cancer arises from apocrine gland-bearing skin cells or as a manifestation of the adjacent primary anal, rectal, or bladder adenocarcinoma. Our patient underwent a full gynecological examination including rectal examination. A biopsy was performed; however, unfortunately, the depth of the invasion could not be identified.

Table 1. Classification of vulvar Paget's disease according to Wilkinson et al. [10]

Primary Vulvar Paget's disease (cutaneous)	Type 1a	Cutaneous vulvar noninvasive Paget's disease
	Type 1b	Cutaneous vulvar invasive disease: dermal invasion by Paget's cells
	Type 1c	Cutaneous vulvar disease as a manifestation of an underlying vulvar adenocarcinoma
Secondary vulvar Paget's disease (noncutaneous)	Type 2	Vulvar Paget's diseaseoriginating from rectal or anal adenocarcinoma
	Type 3	Vulvar Paget's diseaseoriginating from urogenital neoplasia

A large range of interventions, ranging from surgical to noninvasive techniques, are currently available for vulvar Paget's disease. The challenge is how to treat a disease that may not be clinicallyvisible. Edey et al. in 2013 (Cochrane review) performed a thorough systematic search for a scientifically well-informed treatment [11]. However, there is no reliable evidence regarding the intervention for Paget's disease of the vulva. Surgery still remains the primary intervention, although there has been no multicenter, randomized, controlled trial assessing the efficacy of this intervention. Surgery for EMPD mainly comprises wide local excision with or without inguinofemoral lymph node dissection [11]. If an underlying invasive carcinoma is present, it should be treated in a manner similar to that used for treating squamous vulvar cancer. The treatment may require radical vulvectomy and at least an ipsilateralinguinofemoral lymphadenectomy [12]. The surgical margins and the defect after excision are the clinical challenges that may affect the patients' prognosis. Paget cells are difficult to recognize in frozen sections withthe false negative rate ranging from 10% to 13%. However, the relationship between the status of the free marginand recurrence remains unclear. The local recurrence rate after the surgical treatment of vaginal EMPD has been reported to be 34% – 56%, even after utilizing reconstructive skin grafts and flaps. Studies have shown high recurrence rates regardless of the status of the free margin [11].

Radiotherapy is another modality for the treatment of EMPD. Although it has been primarily used as an option for patients who are not eligible for surgery or who decline surgery, there have been no clinical trials assessing its efficacy for the treatment of EMPD. Radiotherapy alone is an alternative therapeutic approach for patients with extensive inoperable disease or medical contraindications. Definitive radiotherapy can be used in elderly patients or patients with medical contraindications [8]. Adjuvant radiotherapy may be considered in the presence of risk factors associated with local recurrence, such as dermal invasion, lymph node metastasis, close or positive surgical margins, perineal tumors, tumors with large diameter, multifocal lesions, extensive disease, the histologic findings of coexisting adenocarcinoma or vulvar carcinoma, high Ki-67 expression, adnexal involvement, or possibly the overexpression of HER-2/neu. Salvage radiotherapy can be usedin patients who exhibit inoperable locoregional recurrence or who decline additional surgery. Recurrence rates following radiotherapy after long-term follow-upsare reported to be <20%. In one study, adjuvant postoperative radiotherapy was administered to 51 patients (55.4%), and 40 patients received radiotherapy as primary treatment. A dose of 40 – 50 Gy is recommended for intraepithelial EMPD and that of 55 – 65 Gy is recommended for invasive EMPD or for an associated adenocarcinoma [8].

CONCLUSION

EMPD is a rare disease involving the skin and apocrine glands of the vulva, anoderm, scrotum, penis, and axilla. Owing to its rare nature, research on available treatment options is difficult. Currently, the standard treatment modality is surgical resection; however, it is associated with a high rate of recurrence. Other treatment options include imiquimod 5% cream, Mohs surgery, radiation therapy, and phototherapy. The success of the treatments varies with each case depends on timing of diagnosis and radicality of surgical treatment. Further investigation regarding this case is needed.

REFERENCES

[1] van der Linden, M.; Meeuwis, K. A.; Bulten, J.; Bosse, T.; van Poelgeest, M. I.; de Hullu, J. A. (2016). Paget disease of the vulva. *Crit. Rev. Oncol. Hematol,* 101:60 - 74.

[2] Anton, C.; Luiz, A. V.; Carvalho, F. M.; Baracat, E. C.; Carvalho, J. P. (2011). Clinical treatment of vulvar Paget's disease: a case report. *Clinics,* (Sao Paulo), 66:1109 - 11.

[3] Paget, J. (1874). On disease of the mammary areola preceding cancer of the mammary gland. St. Bartholemew. *Hosp. Res. Lond*, 10: 87 - 89.

[4] Dubreuilh, W. (1901). Paget's disease of the vulva. *Br. J. Dermatol,* 13: 407 - 13.

[5] Fardal, R. W., Kierland, R. R., Clagett, O. T., Woolner, L. B. (1964). Prognosis in cutaneous Paget's disease. *Postgrad. Med,* 36: 584 - 93.

[6] Chiu, T. W., Wong, P. S., Ahmed, K., Lam, S. C., Ying, S. Y., Burd, A. (2007). Extramammary Paget's disease in Chinese males: a 21-year experience. *World J. Surg,* 31:1941 - 6.

[7] Guerra, R., Misra, S. (2013) Management of Extramammary Paget's Disease: A Case Report and Review of the Literature. *Case Rep. Dermatol. Med*: 436390.

[8] Tolia, M.; Tsoukalas, N.; Sofoudis, C.; Giaginis, C.; Spyropoulou, D.; Kardamakis, D. et al. (2016). Primary extramammary invasive Paget's vulvar disease: what is the standard, what are the challenges and what is the future for radiotherapy? *BMC Cancer,*16: 563.

[9] Onaiwu, C. O., Salcedo, M. P., Pessini, S. A., Munsell, M. F., Euscher, E. E., Reed, K. E. et al. (2017). Paget's disease of the vulva: A review of 89 cases. *Gynecol. Oncol. Rep.,* 19: 46 - 9.

[10] Wilkinson, E. J.; Brown, H. M. (2002). Vulvar Paget disease of urothelial origin: a report of three cases and a proposed classification of vulvar Paget disease. *Hum. Pathol.*, 33:549 - 54.

[11] Edey, K. A., Allan, E., Murdoch, J. B., Cooper, S., Bryant, A. (2013). Interventions for the treatment of Paget's disease of the vulva (Review). *Cochrane Database of Systematic Reviews*.

[12] Hacker, N. F., Eifel, P. J. (2015). Berek and Hacker's *Gynecologic Oncology*. 6th ed. Philadelphia: Wolters Kluwer.

In: Obstetric and Gynecology Case Report ISBN: 978-1-53616-711-5
Editor: Dwiana Ocviyanti

Chapter 25

HOLISTIC MANAGEMENT OF GYNECOLOGICAL CASES IN CIPTO MANGUNKUSUMO HOSPITAL

Dwiana Ocviyanti[1], Kristian Alda[2,*] and Lili Widjaya[2]

[1]Department of Obstetric and Gynaecology,
Faculty of Medicine, Universitas Indonesia,
Dr. Cipto Mangunkusumo Hospital, Jakarta, Indonesia
[2]Faculty of Medicine, Universitas Indonesia, Jakarta, Indonesia

ABSTRACT

Several patients are referred to Dr. Cipto Mangunkusumo National General Hospital due to complicated gynecological problems, both biological and psychological, which affect their life. Therefore, a holistic biopsychosocial treatment should be implemented, which requires interprofessional cooperation. The aim of this study is to present

* Corresponding Author's E-mail: kristianalda@yahoo.com.

gynecological cases requiring holistic treatment and interprofessional management. Seven patients with gynecological problems were admitted to Ciptomangunkusumo General Hospital during 2018 – 2019. The inclusion criteria were gynecological conditions requiring holistic management. Of the seven patients, three had endometriosis, one had adenomyosis, one had Mayer–Rokitansky–Küster–Hauser syndrome, one had fistule vesicovaginal, and one had experienced sexual abuse. These patients were managed in collaboration with other professionals, including pediatricians, psychiatrists, and law experts. Moreover, the patient's family should also be involved in patient management. The conclusion is that in complicated gynecological cases with a high difficulty level, holistic management plays an important role in treatment. An interprofessional approach also plays an important role to increase patients' quality of life.

Keywords: holistic, gynecological case, biopsychosocial aspect, interprofessional management

INTRODUCTION

In Indonesia, some gynecological cases such as mioma uteri, ovary cyst, uterine bleeding, and prolapse uteri, among others, can be found. Gynecological problems limit patients in performing activities of daily activity living. Gynecological patients usually complain of menstrual pain, vaginal bleeding, discharge, burning sensation, and abdominal pain [1]. They usually ignore these symptoms and visit the hospital at the later stage of the disease, leading to late diagnosis and requiring further treatment and referral to a higher health facility. Gynecological patients with conditions that are difficult to manage are referred to Dr. Cipto Mangunkusumo National General Hospital (RSCM) hospital. In addition to having gynecological diseases, these patients present with psychological and social problems.

Therefore, a holistic approach involving the biopsychosocial well-being of patients should be established. The biopsychosocial model looks at the interconnection between biology, psychology, and socioenvironmental factor. The application of biopsychosocial model will give better result in reduce anxiety and improve knowledge of the patient [2]. Along with this model, interprofessional collaboration is also required as part of the treatment.

CASE PRESENTATION

This case series was conducted by obstetrics and gynecology specialists with Dr. Dwiyana Ocviyanti as the adviser. Patients from a teaching hospital affiliated with the University of Indonesia's Faculty of Medicine were recruited in a wide range of times. Patients with gynecological problems who had obtained consent from their family members or those who consented to participate themselves were included in this study.

Case 1: Holistic Handling of Sexually Abused Children

A 15-year-old female patient was brought to the forensic department to undergo a medicolegal examination as she suspected had been sexually abused in their neighborhood.

At first, she denied the sexual harassment to her parents because she received threats from the perpetrator. The perpetrator was a teacher who taught Quran to the victim. The victim has been raped five times already; however, she claimed that only sexual harassment was done, such as opening the victim's clothes, hugging, kissing, and touching the pubic and breast areas. The victim claimed that the perpetrator had never put a finger or genitals into her genitals. On physical examination, no signs of sexual violence were noted and her vital signs and general condition were normal. Gynecological examination revealed no wound on the pubic lips and intact ring-shaped hymen. After forensics examination with the presence of a midwife, the victim was then referred to the psychiatric and pediatric departments.

Case 2: Biopsychosocial Aspects of Patients with Chronic Pelvic Pain Due to Bilateral Endometriosis Cysts with Infertility

A 34-year-old female patient presented with complaints of painful menstruation since 2 years, worsened in the last 2 years. Pain was experienced repeatedly every menstruation. The pain requiring her to take painkiller medication. She also complained of abdominal enlargement since November 2016. She could even palpate a lump in her stomach. She had already been treated at Bajawa General Hospital because of bilateral endometriosis cysts and was advised surgery; however, she was referred to RSCM due to fear of adhesions. The patient has been married for 15 years with a 1-year-old child.

From the physical examination the elastic portion pushed posteriorly, palpable cystic mass in the right adnexa as high as the center, and the cystic mass up to two fingers above the center of the left adnexa. On ultrasound examination, the uterus was anteflexed, with normal shape and size and homogeneous myometrium. The uterine cavity had no abnormal mass. The stratum endometrial basal layer was normal, 9mm thick. The endocervix and portio vaginalis were also normal. Cystic mass was found in both adnexa, which appeared to be bilateral endometriosis cysts. Both ovaries adhere to each other; therefore, she was finally diagnosed with bilateral endometriosis cysts with adnexal attachment. Laboratory tests revealed Ca 125 level of 86.7U/ml and anti-mullerian hormone level of 0.3ng/ml.

The patient was diagnosed with chronic pelvic pain in bilateral endometriosis cysts with internal genital adhesions, and 12 year infertile. Therefore, laparoscopic bilateral cystectomy was performed.

Case 3: Vesicovaginal Fistula in a Primiparous Woman with Prolonged Second Stage of Labor

A 26-year-old primigravida patient arrived with a long second stage of labor for >24h with intrauterine fetal death (IUFD). The patient is aterm with irregular antenatal care. She felt cramp 3 days before presentation, which worsened since 30h ago. The patient was helped by a local shaman but the baby was not yet born. Initially, fetal movement was still observed, but it was no longer felt over time. After 24 h, the patient was referred to the local health center, but was then referred to the hospital due to limited resources. The patient was diagnosed with prolonged second stage of labor in G1 fetal term pregnancy with a single head presentation IUFD. Then, forceps delivery was performed. A 3,400-g IUFD baby girl was delivered with grade III perineal rupture. The patient then came back on day 16 with complaints of inability to hold urine. A positive cough test was performed in the upper vaginal mucosa, and a catheter was inserted through the urethral mouth, and then advanced into the vagina through the anterior wall. The patient was diagnosed with vesico fistula and uretrovaginal in primipara post extraction forceps on day 16 with IUFD infant. The patient and her husband were only married for 1 year. At that time, conferences with the husbands regarding their wife's condition were conducted, so that they would stay with and not blame them. These educational sessions were conducted by gathering all big families and assisted by midwives as mediators and at the same time help explain the patient's condition to their family.

Case 4: Holistic Management of Dysmenorrhea Secondary to Adenomyosis, Bilateral Endometriosis Cysts, Bilateral Hydrosalpinx, and Internal Genital Attachment

A patient was referred for holistic management due to bilateral endometriosis cysts and adenomyosis in P0A1 with planned total bilateral salpingo-oophorectomy hysterectomy. Menstrual pain was observed since 1 year before admission. The initial pain could be ignored, but the last 3 months had been worsen, requiring the patient to take analgetic twice a day for the first 2 days in each period. The patient is currently not sexually active. A palpable abdominal lump was increasing in size since 7 months of SMRS, which was previously diagnosed as possibly malignant. She had plans to remarry and have children. She was conservatively treated with 1 × 1 tablet of progesterone hormonal derivative therapy along with nonsteroidal anti-inflammatory drug administration and was followed up for 3 months.

She complained of dizziness, and the cost of drug became a burden; therefore, she planned to undergo total bilateral salpingo-oophorectomy hysterectomy. The patient was then informed that her current condition did not allow her to bear children.

Case 5: Aggressive Management of Low-Risk Endometrial Cancer in an Infertile Patient with Low Socioeconomic Status

A 29-year-old patient was referred with endometrial cancer. She had a history of 2.5 months of vaginal bleeding. The obtained specimen showed good differentiation of endometrioid carcinoma. Therefore, she was treated with progressin 600mg/day and evaluated every 3 months.

One year before admission, the patient was referred to RSCM because of amenorrhea for 2 months. The patient was then treated with Yaz 1 × 1 and Metformin 3 × 500mg.

Hysteroscopic resection was performed, and atypical squamous metaplasia was observed. Subsequent examination with magnetic resonance imaging showed endometrial thickening with diffuse restriction that infiltrated the myometrium in the left posterior uterine fundus. Hysteroscopy showed that the endometrium was highly influenced by progesterone without malignancy. Therefore, the patient was diagnosed with 1A endometrial cancer with conservative therapy. Ecamination with immunohistochemistry to assess mismatch repair in several genes such as MSH2, MLH1, MSH6, and PMS2. There are positive results on secondary protein MSH6 were associated with mismatch repair mutations. Ultrasound examination shows an ecogenic period with an irregular edge measuring 14 × 9mm from the endometrial mass. Because hysteroscopy did not show a significant improvement in the patient's condition, a total hysterectomy was performed with left salpingo-oophorectomy.

Case 6: Biopsychosocial Approach in a Woman with Chronic Pelvic Pain, Abnormal Uterine Bleeding, and Primary Subfertility Due to Endometriosis

A 31-year-old patient presented with primary complaints of pelvic pain (VAS 6), anemia due to abnormal uterine bleeding, and primary infertility for 6 years. Two weeks after admission, the patient experienced vaginal bleeding and underwent two blood transfusions within 4 months. She experienced pain during period for 10 years and worsen in the last 2 years. She was taking her medications in the last 6 months; however, she stopped taking them regularly in the last 3 months. She had never undergone any surgery, had not been pregnant, and never had her condition checked by a doctor. She was more worried about the pain than infertility. She was a household assistant, but has recently stopped working because of the pain.

Case 7: Primary Amenorrhea Caused by Mayer–Rokitansky–Küster–Hauser Syndrome

An 18-year-old patient presented with complaints of never having menstruation. The patient also did not have a right kidney and the size of her uterus was said to be small. The patient's breasts started to grow at the age of 11 years. The patient has never been married and has never had sexual relations. She is the third child of three siblings, both of them are males, and no similar family history has been reported. Her physical examination and general status were good within limit. A ribbon-like mass located in the uterus was detected, and other examinations showed normal results. Transrectal ultrasound examination found an exogenous material extending laterally, which originated from a genital band that ends in a cornu form with dysgenesis. Both ovaries were small with antral follicles. The right kidney was not detected. The patient was diagnosed with Mayer–Rokitansky–Küster–Hauser suspected due to primary amenorrhea. Karyotyping and explanation of the disease were performed, and a neovagine reconstruction will be implemented if the patient plans to marry.

DISCUSSION

Holistic management in gynecological patients consists of biological, psychological, social, and cultural aspects [3]. The seven patients presented with different biological problems such as chronic pelvic pain in endometriosis cysts, vesicovaginal fistulae, adenomyosis, endometrial cancer, and endometriosis. Their respective biological problems were managed appropriately.

Psychological problems occurring in gynecological patients include severe pain during menstruation, anxiety for not bearing children, fears of enlarged lumps, and fear about the disease.

In the first case, the patient may worry that she is no longer a virgin, has pubic anatomical damage, and fears the parents' response. The act of sexual harassment in children certainly has an emotional and physical impact. Children who were victims of abuse have the potential to experience stress, depression, and mental shock. They can also experience fear to connect with other people. The long-term effects of sexual harassment are potential phobias for sexual relations when the child reaches adulthood. Therefore, psychological management is very important in sexually abused children. Based on Law Number 23 of 2002 concerning child protection, children as victims have the right to receive rehabilitation from the institution. Rehabilitation is a process of integrated recovery activities, both physical and mental [2, 3]. We learn from this case the management of these patients requires cooperation from law enforcement, family, schools and psychiatrists [4, 5, 6].

The two patients with chronic pelvic pain will certainly experience psychological problems, as pain is a major concern in patients with endometriosis patients. Pelvic pain can affect various aspects of life, such as sleep, eating, and performance of activities of daily living. In 2004, the American College of Obstetrics and Gynecology defined chronic pelvic pain as a cyclical pain occurring at least 6 months that affects the patients' daily activity and thus requiring medical intervention [7]. In our patients, pelvic pain causes anxiety during menstruation. Six patients with chronic pelvic pain also had a psychological impact, i.e., depression. The psychological impact of pelvic pain can be managed in several ways, such as good counseling, and patients must be taught how to manage their pain. In addition, family support will increase the patient's confidence and accept her condition. Patient's acceptance is very important in cases of chronic pelvic pain because of the need to take medications until menopause; thus, disease acceptance can increase compliance with the patient's medication [8, 9].

Another problem that may psychologically affect patients is fear of inability to produce child. A study showed that infertile females are reported to have personal stress and higher social stress than males. In the second case, patients together with their family experience difficulties in accepting the fact that they can no longer produce child. This social problem with the family is certainly a cause of stress. Besides the disease, treatment procedures can also cause infertility. A study analyzed the relationship between hysterectomy and depression in women. This study shows that patients who underwent hysterectomy have depression and anxiety levels two times higher than those who did not. Therefore, infertile patients should be understood and the family should also accept the patient's condition [10, 11].

Enlarged lumps are also one of the problems often experienced by gynecological patients. As in the 4th case, the patient had an abdominal lump, which is feared to progress into a malignant cancer, whereas in the second case, the patient opted for a surgery for the abdominal lump to prevent it from increasing in size and becoming malignant. A study indicated that cancer patients feel hopeless because their disease cannot be prevented anymore. Freud's theory indicated that one hopes to live forever subconsciously, whereas patients with cancer expect an inevitable death. This causes a sense of frustration which over time will become depression, even causing suicide. Spiritual life has an important role in dealing with life-threatening diseases such as cancer. Family and friends' reactions to the physical changes experienced by women during chemotherapy also play an important role in helping people face their illness. Moreover, detailed patient education is also important, as observed in four patients who experienced excessive anxiety, who became calmer after a more detailed explanation of the disease has been provided [12, 13].

Besides psychology, the patients' social aspect should also be considered in gynecological patients, for example, the patient's relationship with her husband. Research shows that patients with gynecological problems have sex fewer times than those without symptoms. This will potentially cause problems in family relationships; therefore, the patient's partner should be also educated on the patient's disease. Patients also can have problems with their social environment, as in case number three. For fear that patients will be considered strange by their environment when using a catheter, we work with local health workers to educate the public.

Conclusion

Holistic management is required for the management of gynecological cases to improve service quality.

References

[1] Gynecological complaints and their associated factors among women in a family health-care clinic.

[2] Edozien, L. C. (2015). Beyond biology: the biopsychosocial model and its application in obstetrics and gynaecology. *BJOG,* 122: 900 - 903.

[3] Borrell-Carrió, F., Suchman, A. L., and Epstein, R. M. (2004). The biopsychosocial model 25 years later: principles, practice, and scientific inquiry. *Annals of Family Medicine*, 2 (6): 576 - 582.

[4] Noviana, I. (2015). Child sexual abuse: Impact and Handling. *Sosio Informa,* 01(1):13 - 28.

[5] Lesmana, C. B., Suryani, L. K., and Tiliopoulos, N. (2015). Cultural considerations in the treatment of mental illness among sexually

abused children and adolescents: the case of Bali, Indonesia. *New Dir. Child Adolesc.*, 147:109 - 16.

[6] Christensen, L. S. (2018). Professionals' perceptions of female child sexual offenders. *Journal of Interpersonal Violence*, 1:886260518785377.

[7] Howard, F. M. (2009). Endometriosis and mechanisms of pelvic pain. *Journal of Minimally Invasive Gynecology*, 16(5): 540 - 50.

[8] Ballweg, M. L. (2004). Impact of endometriosis on women's health: comparative historical data show that the earlier the onset, the more severe the disease. *Best Practice and Research Clinical Obstetrics and Gynaecology*, 18(2): 201 - 18.

[9] Daniels, J. P. and Khan, K. S. (2010). Chronic pelvic pain in woman. *British Medical Journal*, 341: c4834.

[10] Callan, V. J. and Hennessey, J. F. (1989). Strategies for coping with infertility. *British Journal of Medical Psychology*, 62: 343 - 354.

[11] Watkins, J. K. and Baldo, T. D. (2004). The infertility experience: biophsychosocial effects and suggestions for counselor. *Journal of Counseling and Development,* 82: 394.

[12] Sengül, Y. and Ayaz, S. (2016). Psychological problems experienced by women with gynecological cancer and how they cope with it: a phenomenological study in Turkey. *Health and Social Work,* 41: 173 - 181.

[13] Grimm, D., Hasenburg, A., Eulenburg, C., Steinsiek, L., Mayer, S., Eltrop, S., Prieske, K., Trillsch, F., Mahner, S. and Woelber, L. (2015). Sexual activity and function in patients with gynecological malignancies after completed treatment. *Int. J. Gynecol. Cancer*, 25: 1134 - 1141.

In: Obstetric and Gynecology Case Report ISBN: 978-1-53616-711-5
Editor: Dwiana Ocviyanti

Chapter 26

DIAGNOSTIC APPROACH AND SUCCESSFUL MANAGEMENT OF CERVICAL TUBERCULOSIS: A CASE REPORT

Junita Indarti[1,*], Hartono Tjahjadi[2], Ujainah Zaini[3], July Kumalawati[4], Yulia Rosa Saharman[5], Amanda Mustika Sari[1], Andri[1], Caroline Gladys[1], Febian Nathania[1], Adly Nanda Al Fattah[1] and Muhammad Saiful Rizal[1]

[1]Department of Obstetric and Gynecology, Faculty of Medicine, Universitas Indonesia, Dr. Cipto Mangunkusumo Hospital, Jakarta, Indonesia

[2]Department of Pathology Anatomy, Faculty of Medicine, Universitas Indonesia, Dr. Cipto Mangunkusumo Hospital, Jakarta, Indonesia

---

* Corresponding Author's E-mail: junita_indarti@yahoo.com.

[3]Department of Interna Medicine, Faculty of Medicine, Universitas Indonesia, Dr. Cipto Mangunkusumo Hospital, Jakarta, Indonesia
[4]Department of Clinical Pathology, Faculty of Medicine, Universitas Indonesia, Dr. Cipto Mangunkusumo Hospital, Jakarta, Indonesia
[5]Department of Microbiology, Universitas Indonesia, Jakarta, Indonesia

Abstract

Only a few cases of cervical tuberculosis were reported in the literature, making it a rare condition. Additionally, the history and cervical characteristics of cervical tuberculosis resemble those of invasive cervical cancer. A 31-year-old nulliparous woman complained of having vaginal discharge and post-coital bleeding for 1 year prior to admission. The cervical examination revealed an irregular and fragile cervical mass that bled easily. The Pap smear test also suggests atypical squamous cell cannot exclude high-grade squamous intraepithelial lesion (ASCH). A suspected cervical cancer mass was visualized on our colposcopy view. A cervical mass biopsy revealed a chronic granulomatous cervicitis that is probably caused by tuberculous infection. Additionally, the serum interferon-gamma release assay (IGRA) test was positive. Therefore, the patient's clinical and histopathologic diagnosis was cervical tuberculosis. A 4-week administration of first-line antituberculosis treatment resulted in the improvement of the cervical lesion. Based on the clinical and histopathological findings, our patient was diagnosed with cervical tuberculosis. First-line antituberculosis drugs are the treatment of choice for cervical tuberculosis.

Keywords: diagnosis, cervical tuberculosis, management

Introduction

Cervical tuberculosis is a rare form of extragenital tuberculosis. It attributes to 0.1%–0.65% of all cases of tuberculosis and 5%–24% of all cases of genital tract tuberculosis [1]. Both hematogenous or lymphatic dissemination and direct extension play an important role in the pathogenesis of cervical tuberculosis [2]. Reportedly, the use of sputum as a sexual lubricant may be a transmission route of *Mycobacterium tuberculosis* [3]. Further, the diagnostic approach of cervical tuberculosis is clinically challenging because it can be easily misdiagnosed as cervical malignancy [1]. Furthermore, specific management guidelines in treating cervical tuberculosis have yet to be published in the literature. We present our complete approach for the diagnosis, development of cervical tuberculosis, and successful management.

CASE ILLUSTRATION

A 31-year-old nulliparous woman complained of having vaginal discharge and post-coital bleeding for 1 year. The patient had a history of 2-year primary infertility. She had a regular period. She denied any history of chronic cough, night sweating, significant weight loss, immunodeficiency diseases, immunosuppressant medications, or personal or family exposure to tuberculosis. However, she had a history of intestinal tuberculosis for which she completed first-line therapy 10 years prior. Her first sexual intercourse occurred at the age of 17. She had no family history of a gynecologic malignancy, she did not smoke, and she had no remarkable past medical history.

Physical examination, the patient had no palpable supraclavicular or inguinal lymph nodes.Direct visual examination of the cervix revealed an abnormal cervical appearance with a fragile and irregular cervical mass that bled easily. On transvaginal ultrasound, we found an 11-mm endocervical polyp, with regular endometrial basal layer, and ovaries of normal appearance (Figure 1). Pap smear analysis showed atypical squamous cells of undetermined significance (ASC-US). Colposcopic examination revealed a mass with an irregular surface, increasing vascularity, and mild acetowhite changes (Figure 2). Thus, the patient was suspected to have invasive cervical cancer. She underwent a large loop excision of the transformation zone (LLETZ). Histopathological examination of the sample revealed granulomatous chronic cervicitis without caseous necrotized stroma that could possibly be caused by tuberculous infection (Figure 3).

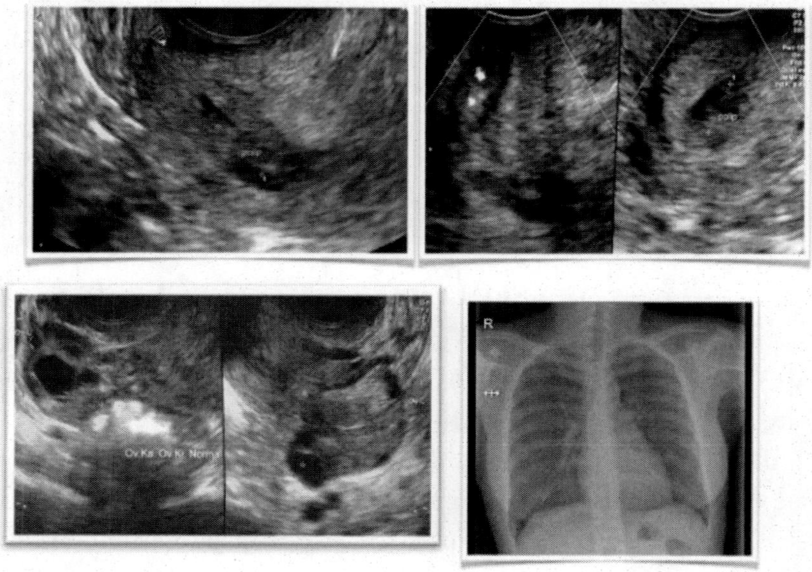

Figure 1. Transvaginal ultrasound revealed an 11-mm endocervical polyp (upper left and right), ovaries of normal appearance (lower left), and normal findings in a chest radiograph (lower right).

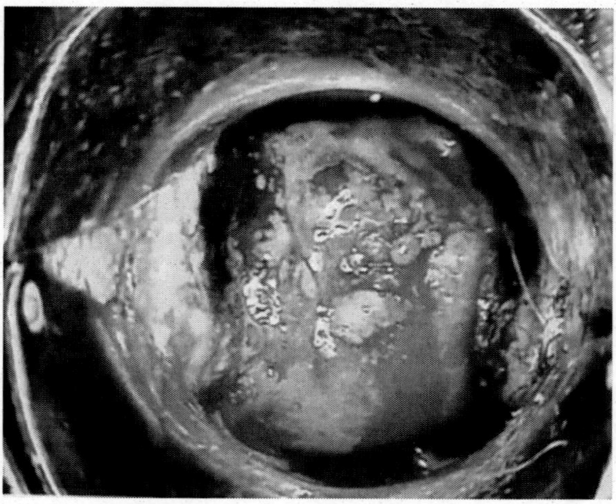

Figure 2. Colposcopic examination revealed a mass with irregular surface, increasing vascularity, and mild acetowhite changes.

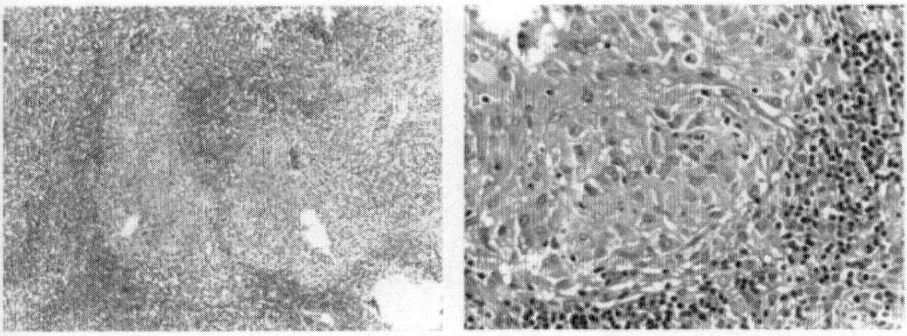

Figure 3. Pathological examination of a hematoxylin–eosin stained sample of a cervical biopsy. Chronic granulomatous cervicitis (left, original magnification ×10) with several epithelioid cells (right, original magnification, ×40) that were caused by tuberculosis.

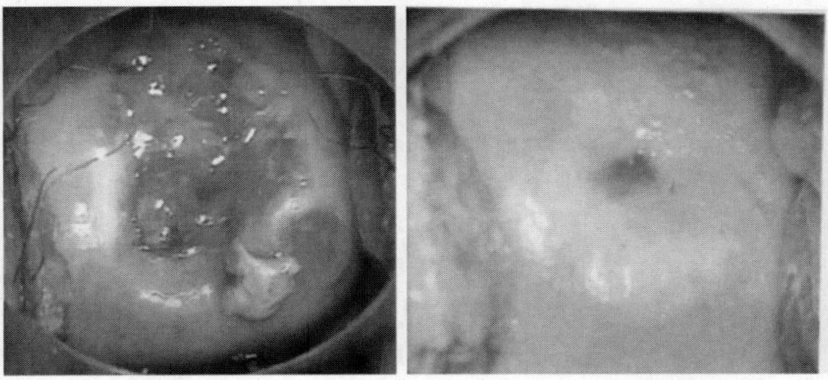

Figure 4. Cervical appearance on colposcopic view before (left) and 4 weeks after (right) antituberculosis treatment.

Two weeks after the LLETZ procedure and under colposcopic view, a vaginal swab and abnormal tissue sampling were obtained. The specimens were sent for microbiological culture. Ziehl–Neelsen staining found no acid-resistant bacteria. Additionally, the chest radiograph showed a normal appearance of both lungs. The patient's sputum was negative for acid-fast bacillus (AFB). However, the patient tested positive in the interferon-gamma release assay (IGRA) test.

First-line antituberculosis drugs was prescribed as the treatment of choice. The regimen included isoniazid (5 mg/kgBW), rifampicin (10 mg/kgBW), pyrazinamide (25 mg/kgBW), and ethambutol (15 mg/kgBW) for 2 months. Treatment with isoniazid (5 mg/BW) and rifampicin (10 mg/BW) was continued for 7 months. During the initial 4-week treatment, improvement of cervical lesions was already apparent (Figure 4).

DISCUSSION

The burden of tuberculosis in Indonesia is among the highest in the world. There were 1,020,000 estimated cases of new active tuberculosis in 2017, with an incidence of approximately 395 per 100.000 population. Indonesia has the second highest number of new tuberculosis cases in the world. In fact, 60% of the new cases mainly emerge in six countries: India, Indonesia, China, Nigeria, Pakistan, and South Africa [1,2]. There were an estimated 9.4 million extrapulmonary tuberculosis (EPTB) cases worldwide in 2009; thus, EPTB remains a concern. EPTB mainly includes tuberculous lymphadenitis and pericarditis, as well as pleural, skeletal, central nervous system, abdominal, and genitourinary TB [4]. Fallopian tubes and ovaries are commonly involved in genital tuberculosis [3]. Nevertheless, cervical tuberculosis attributes only to 0.1%–0.65% of all tuberculosis cases. It is possible that the roles of the stratified squamous epithelium of the ectocervix and cervical mucus are useful in preventing bacterial penetration [5].

In this particular case, the previous EPTB infection (intestinal tuberculosis) and the habit of using sputum as the sexual lubricant could be considered risk factors of tuberculosis. The finding of chronic granulomatous inflammation was a pathognomonic feature of tuberculosis which led to the diagnosis of cervical tuberculosis in this patient. This histopathological finding is common in cases of chronic infection caused by *Mycobacterium tuberculosis* complexes, such as *M. tuberculosis*, *M. canettii*, *M. africanum*, *M. bovis*, *M. microti*, *M. pinnipedii*, *and M. caprae*. Predisposing factors for tuberculosis include those that affect the patient's immunity, for example, poverty, overcrowding with improper ventilation, inadequate access to health care, malnutrition, diabetes mellitus, smoking, alcohol and/or drug abuse, end-stage renal disease, cancer treatment, haemodialysis, and HIV infection. However, our patient had no tuberculosis-specific risk factors [6].

Tuberculosis develops as a result of direct bacterial invasion to any bodily organ or abnormal immune reactions secondary to mycobacterial products. Tubercle bacilli are able to remain dormant in tissues and persist for many years. With primary tuberculosis, microorganisms are disseminated through the bloodstream to other organs, where they remain dormant in latent foci. In 5%–15% of infected patients, these dormant foci break down (liquefaction necrosis and cavitation), causing dispersion of the tubercle bacilli [6]. This condition could be found through histopathological examination. Chronic granulomatous cervicitis without caseous necrotized stroma could be induced by a tuberculous infection.

Secondary disease, or reactivation tuberculosis, occurs as a consequence of decreased cellular immunity. Genitourinary tuberculosis is usually caused by reactivation of these dormant organisms, within the first 2 years following the primary infection by *M. tuberculosis* (90%–95%) and very rarely (5%–10%) by *M. bovis* [6]. It is fairly common that genital tuberculosis occurs a result of reactivation of latent foci in other organs [1]. The first mechanism of transmission is the hematogenous route from any of the primary sites, which accounts for about 90% of the cases. The second mechanism is direct descending spread or lymphatic spread directly from infected organs, such as the bowel or mesenteries. The third mechanism consists of a direct extension to the genital tract organs from the tuberculous abdominal viscera. The latter is the ascending infection, which could manifest as a vulvar, vaginal, and/or cervical lesion. The risk for transmission of this patient increased due to the use of sputum as a sexual lubricant. Although rare, sexual transmission has been reported, as 3.9% of men with genitourinary tuberculosis can harbor bacilli in their semen. Therefore, tuberculosis screening via chest radiograph and sputum AFB was also planned for the patient's husband in order to evaluate possible transmission mechanisms, such as the ascending or direct infection that possibly occurred during sexual intercourse [5, 6, 7].

It is possible for primary cervical tuberculosis to be transmitted by the sexual partner during intercourse. Further, it is possible for woman who had dormant tuberculosis in another organ and excreted tubercle bacilli in her stool, urine, or sputum to develop secondary cervical tuberculosis. If such bodily fluids come into contact with microabrasions in the skin or mucosa of the genitalia, it may lead to genital tuberculosis. Cervical tuberculosis could also affect the internal reproductive organs, including the fallopian tubes, endometrium, and ovaries. The fallopian tubes can become congested and occupied by military tubercles, whereas the endometrium present caseation and ulceration (in 50%–80% of cases), which can lead to intrauterine adhesions (2.5%). Furthermore, ovaries develop into tubo-ovarian masses (in 20%–30% of cases) [5, 6]. Thus, women with cervical tuberculosis may have fertility issues resulting from the involvement of internal reproductive organs.

Approximately 11% of patients are asymptomatic. However, cervical tuberculosis may cause chronic pelvic pain, dysmenorrhea, dyspareunia, and amenorrhea. Other symptoms, such as vaginal discharge and tubo-ovarian mass with ascites, can also be found. Nevertheless, physical examination may be normal in up to 50% of cases. In a general examination, the patient can appear poorly nourished and have fever, enlargement of the cervical lymph nodes, and signs of pulmonary tuberculosis. During abdominal examination, the abdomen can feel doughy upon palpation, which suggests peritoneal tuberculosis, or it could be distended due to ascites. During pelvic examination, frozen pelvis could be present due to adhesions and restricted mobility of the uterus. Signs such as adnexal mass (i.e., tubo-ovarian mass or hydrosalpinx), enlarged uterus secondary to pyometra, and tenderness in the pouch of Douglas or to cervical movement have also been reported. It is necessary to differentiate between cervical cancer and cervical tuberculosis by cervical biopsy [8].

Early diagnosis of EPTB is essential for further treatment and control of this infectious disease. However, low bacterium detection rate and difficult access to pathological evidence can make the diagnosis of EPTB more elusive than that of pulmonary tuberculosis. The tuberculin skin test (TST), using the Mantoux method, has been extensively used as a diagnostic test for tuberculosis, although its specificity and sensitivity are quite low. As an alternative to TST, IGRA, a T-cell-based test, has been developed. IGRA may have a slight advantage over TST in detecting latent tuberculosis infection. It uses tuberculosis-specific antigens, which are expected to increase the tests sensitivity and specifity [4, 9]. The sensitivity and positive predictive value of IGRA are 87.7% and 83.3%, respectively. Meanwhile, the specificity is low at 63%, indicating that a negative IGRA result does not exclude the possibility of harboring extrapulmonary TB [10].

Nowadays, diagnosing both active and latent tuberculous infection remains to be a major challenge because both TST and IGRA cannot differentiate between active and latent tuberculosis infection. Culture results are generally unsatisfactory. It is difficult to establish the diagnoses of active tuberculosis. In latent infection, the diagnosis is also difficult due to lack of gold standard [4, 9].

EPTB is usually difficult to diagnose due to unspecific symptoms, and the acid-fast bacilli smear and culture from tissue and body fluid often yield negative results. Therefore, diagnosing EPTB should not only be based on IGRA or TST result alone but should include epidemiologic considerations and medical history as well as other clinical information. Additionally, the invasive procedures are usually required for histopathological diagnosis [10, 11].

Cervical tuberculosis is diagnosed by histological examination from a biopsy of the cervical tissue. The image of typical granulomata can be used for the diagnosis, but the gold standard for diagnosis is the isolation of the *Mycobacterium*. Culture and staining for acid-fast bacilli may not be useful because in roughly a third of cases, these evaluations yield negative results. An alternative test that can be used to detect tuberculosis infection is the molecular tuberculosis test (Xpert MTB/RIF) enzyme-linked immunosorbent assay and polymerase chain reaction [5, 12].

Additionally, HIV testing should be performed in patients because sometimes, cervical tuberculosis is associated with HIV infection. Hence, our patient was tested in order to rule out sexually transmitted diseases, such as TPHA, VDRL, and HIV. Fortunately, the results were negative. Further, the differential diagnosis for granulomatous diseases of the cervix includes amoebiasis, schistosomiasis, brucellosis, tularemia, sarcoidosis, and foreign body reaction [12].

Our patient did not present any signs of active pulmonary tuberculosis. History of intestinal tuberculosis 10 years earlier, family history of TB exposure, positive IGRA assessment, and histologically confirmed granulomatous cervicitis possibly induced by tuberculous infection further support the diagnosis of cervical tuberculosis. The IGRA test alone is not specific for diagnosing latent tuberculous infection. Based on the course of the disease, latent tuberculous infection could have possibly occurred in our patient. However, direct contact infection through the sputum during sexual intercourse could possibly increase the risk of cervical tuberculosis in the patient.

Cervical tuberculosis is one of the rare forms of EPTB. We found no specific clinical trial or guideline for the treatment of cervical tuberculosis. INDEX-TB guideline panels stated that a 6-month treatment with a first-line regimen of antituberculosis drugs is recommended for abdominal tuberculosis [13]. Based on the treatment administered to our patient, first-line antituberculosis drugs resulted in favorable outcomes for cervical tuberculosis. However, the source of the tuberculous infection should also be treated in a comprehensive way.

Conclusion

The diagnosis of cervical tuberculosis is challenging. In the case presented here, the history and cervical characteristics of cervical tuberculosis resemble those of invasive cervical cancer. However, it was possible to diagnose cervical tuberculosis in our patient based on clinical and histopathological examination. First-line treatment with antituberculosis drugs resulted in improved cervical lesion in our patient.

Cervical tuberculosis presents a complex scenario; thus, multi-disciplinary expertise should be involved for appropriate diagnosis and management. The diagnosis of cervical tuberculosis should be listed as part of the differential diagnosis of post-coital bleeding and abnormal cervical lesions, especially in Indonesia, a country considered to be one of the major contributors to the worldwide incidence of tuberculosis [14]. It is likely that the lack of prospective randomized treatment studies, and therefore, objective data, has prevented the development of clinical guidelines for the treatment of cervical tuberculosis.

REFERENCES

[1] World Health Organization. (2017). *Global Tuberculosis Report*. In: World Health Organization, editor. Geneva; Switzerland

[2] Collins, D; Hafidz, F; Mustikawati, D. (2017). The economic burden of tuberculosis in Indonesia. *The international journal of tuberculosis and lung disease*, 21:1041-1048.

[3] Lamba, H; Byrne, M; Goldin, R; Jenkins, C. (2002). Tuberculosis of the cervix: case presentation and a review of the literature. *Sexually transmitted infections*, 78: 62-63.

[4] Fan, L.; Chen, Z.; Hao, XH; Hu, ZY; Xiao, HP. (2012). Interferon-gamma release assays for the diagnosis of extrapulmonary tuberculosis: a systematic review and meta-analysis. FEMS: *Immunology & Medical Microbiology*, 65: 456-466.

[5] Elkattan, E AM; Hettow, H; Hussein, E; Assaad, J. (2014). Tuberculous cervicitis mimicking cancer cervix: A case study. *Middle East Fertility Society Journal*, 19: 75-77.

[6] Thejavathy, GV. (2017). Aetiopathogenesis of Female Genital Tuberculosis In: Shela CN SK; editor. *Female Genital Tuberculosis.* Bengaluru: BSOG Focus: 3-5.

[7] Singh, S; Gupta, V; Modi, S; Rana, P; Duhan, A; Sen, R. (2010). Tuberculosis of uterine cervix: a report of two cases with variable clinical presentation. *Tropical Doctor,* 40: 125-126.

[8] Nagawathnamma, R. (2017). Clinical Features of Genital Tuberculosis. In: Sheela N. SK; editor. Female Genital Tuberculosis. *Bengalaru: BSOG Focus*: 6-8.

[9] Adilistya, T. (2016). The benefits of interferon-gamma release assay examination for the diagnosis of tuberculosis in Indonesia. *CDK, 242.* (43): 545-550.

[10] Rumende, CM; Hadi, EJ; Tanjung, G; Saputri, IN; Sasongko, R. (2018). The benefit of interferon-gamma release assay for diagnosis of extrapulmonary tuberculosis. *Acta medica Indonesiana*, 50:138-143.

[11] Gupta, B; Shree, S; Rajaram, S; Goel, N. (2016). Genital tuberculosis: Unusual presentations. *International Journal of Mycobacteriology*, 5:357-359.

[12] CDC. (2010). Morbidity and mortality weekly report. *Updated guidelines for using interferon-gamma release assays to detect Mycobacterium tuberculous infection–United States*:59.

[13] Sharma, S. K., Ryan, H., Khaparde, S., Sachdeva, KS, Singh, AD; Mohan, A, Sarin, R, Paramasivan, CN, Kumar, P, Nischal, N, Khatiwada, S., Garner, P., Tharyan, P. (2017). Index-TB guidelines: Guidelines on extrapulmonary tuberculosis for India. *Indian Journal of Medical Research*, 145: 448-463.

[14] *Global tuberculosis report. (2017).* Geneva: World Health Organization; Licence: CC BY-NC- SA 3.0 IGO.

About the Editor

Dr. Dwiana Ocviyanti, SpOG (K) MPH
Faculty of Medicine, Universitas Indonesia,
Dr. Cipto Mangunkusumo Hospital, Jakarta, Indonesia
E-mail: drliliwidjaya10@gmail.com.

Dwiana Ocviyanti, an Obstetricians & Gynecologist, works as an educational staff in the Department of Obstetric & Gynecology, Faculty of Medicine Universitas Indonesia-Cipto Mangunkusumo Hospital Jakarta, Indonesia. She graduated as a medical doctor from Universitas Indonesia. She also got a doctoral degree in Epidemiology from Faculty of Public Health Universitas Indonesia and a master degree in Public Health from Faculty of Medicine Universitas Gajah Mada. She finished her training in Obstetric & Gynecology in Faculty of Medicine Universitas Indonesia-Cipto Mangunkusumo Hospital Jakarta. Currently she is a Deputy Editor-in-Chief of Indonesian Journal of Obstetrics and Gynecology (INAJOG) and Editor-in-Chief Journal of The Indonesian Medical Association (JINMA).

Her research has been published in approximately 13 national and international journals in the past three years.

INDEX

D

E

F

G

H

I

L

M

N

O

Related Nova Publications

Immune System Dominant Role in Tissue Homeostasis, Neo-Oogenesis, Regenerative Medicine, and Cancer Growth and Treatment

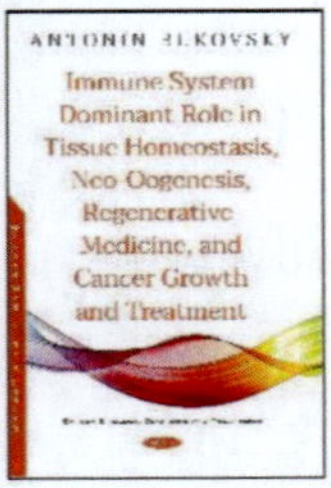

Author: Antonin Bukovsky

Series: Obstetrics and Gynecology Advances

Book Description: The dominant role of the immune system in managing homeostasis of distinct normal tissues and in stimulating cancer growth in regenerative medicine for gonadal infertility and aging diseases, effective immunotherapy without adverse events of inoperable epithelial ovarian cancers (EOCs), and long-lasting cancer immune prophylaxis are reported.

eBook ISBN: 978-1-53615-488-7
Retail Price: $82

Pelvic Inflammatory Disease

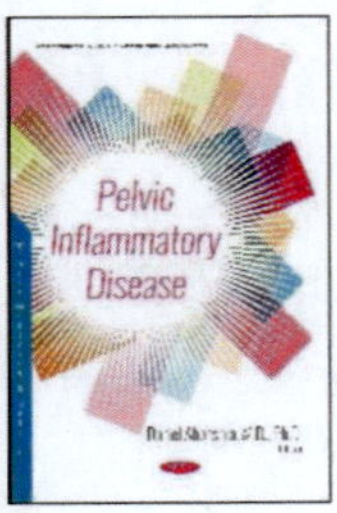

Editor: Daniel Abehsera

Series: Obstetrics and Gynecology Advances

Book Description: Pelvic inflammatory disease (PID) is an entity whose diagnosis is not always easy. The PID comprises a wide range of clinical forms ranging from banal to severe disease processes that compromise the life of the patient.

Softcover ISBN: 978-1-53615-193-0
Retail Price: $82

To see a complete list of Nova publications, please visit our website at www.novapublishers.com

Related Nova Publications

Breast Surgery: Indications and Techniques

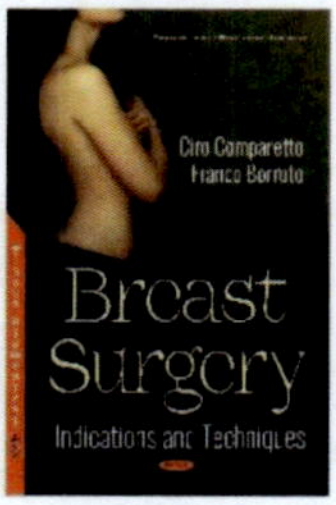

Authors: Ciro Comparetto and Franco Borruto

Series: Obstetrics and Gynecology Advances

Book Description: Breast surgery is the surgical treatment of breast diseases. Its fields of application are particularly breast cancer therapy and the plastic-reconstructive time that follows.

Hardcover ISBN: 978-1-53613-489-6
Retail Price: $230

Postpartum Hemorrhage and Cesarean Section: Complications of Labor and Delivery

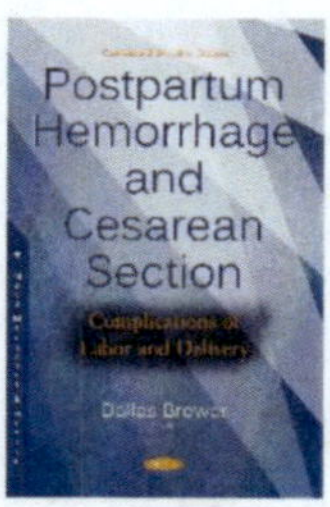

Editor: Dallas Brewer

Series: Obstetrics and Gynecology Advances

Book Description: In this collection, a combined method of preventing and stopping a postpartum obstetric hemorrhage is proposed, involving surgical hemostasis by ligation of the descending branch of the uterine artery and placement of a hemostatic external supraplacental pleated suture.

Softcover ISBN: 978-1-53614-000-2
Retail Price: $82

To see a complete list of Nova publications, please visit our website at www.novapublishers.com